ONE DOCTOR'S ODYSSEY
THE SOCIAL LESION

The Memoirs of
Sir Donald Acheson

Published 2007 by arima publishing

www.arimapublishing.com

ISBN 978-1-84549-276-2

Printed and bound in the United Kingdom

Typeset in Palatino Linotype 11/14

Abramis is an imprint of arima publishing

arima publishing
ASK House, Northgate Avenue
Bury St Edmunds, Suffolk IP32 6BB
t: (+44) 01284 700321

www.arimapublishing.com

This book is dedicated to the members of WHO, UNHCR, the British and International Red Cross, The Red Crescent, the brave fliers in the airlift, and other voluntary organisations who worked to reduce the suffering of the citizens of the Former Yugoslavia and the Russian Republics adjoining the Caspian Sea during the disturbances of the 1990s.

FOREWORD

The Right Honourable Norman Fowler

The Chief Medical Officer is an adviser at the very top of Government. Health Ministers are rarely medically qualified – any more than Defence Ministers have had long armed service careers. The result is that the CMO is required to advise the Government on everything from salmonella in eggs, to HIV/AIDS. It was in dealing with this last challenge that I worked most closely with Donald Acheson.

I was Secretary of State for Health (and indeed Social Security) for six years between 1981 and 1987. For the bulk of that time Donald Acheson was my chief medical adviser. Together we faced public health problems like a food poisoning outbreak in a northern hospital which killed more than 20 old people, as well as other issues which were intensely political. One of these was our battle with the pharmaceutical industry and extraordinarily the BMA, to substitute generic drugs for some brand products at an enormous saving to the Health Service. The policy was never reversed.

But it was on HIV/AIDS that we worked most closely. It needs to be remembered that in the mid-1980s this was a new threat. There were no familiar signposts. The nearest equivalent was the way we tackled venereal disease in the two world wars. We decided that the best policy was to be entirely frank with the British public and to tell them (using television advertising and bill-boards) that there was no cure and no vaccine. The only course open was prevention which required reducing the exchange of sexual partners and the use of condoms.

At the time we were much criticised for the course we took. We were told it was a "moral" issue and the Government should not interfere. We were told that our prevention advice made matters worse by extending knowledge to young people. We were told to isolate AIDS sufferers. We did not follow that advice. Instead we sent leaflets to every household and introduced measures like free needle exchanges for drug users and making condoms widely available. The result was that Britain had one of the lowest figures for infection in Europe and substantially less than the United States, who at the time took a much more *laissez-faire* approach.

Donald Acheson played a vital part in the battle against HIV/AIDS but, as his book shows, he achieved much more. He writes movingly, for example, of his experiences in what was once Yugoslavia and the dreadful effects of ethnic cleansing. He also describes his early life and his father's work with the Royal Army Medical Corps in the First World War.

It is a fascinating memoir which for me underlines one central point. We are amazingly fortunate to have public servants of the quality of Donald Acheson working for our good.

The Right Honourable Norman Fowler

PREFACE

The Social Lesion defined:

"A 'social lesion' exists when one group in a society regards itself as inalienably superior to another hence engendering a sense of disadvantage, loss of control and frustration in the latter" as occurs in Ulster, The Black Sea area of Russia and Bosnia.

Lecture: "The origins of Civil Unrest"
Given by Sir Donald Acheson at the Fort Mason Centre, San Francisco, California 28/4/99

Contents

List of Illustrations

1. Sir Donald Acheson
2. Factors underlying cohesion into groups race, religion, culture, tribe
3. Siege of Sarajevo – despair
4. Ethnic cleansing by destroying homes
5. Risto Tervahauta
6. Displaced families
7. Sarajevo – uncollected rubbish
8. Prisoners of war being kept in deplorable conditions in flagrant violation of the Geneva Convention
9. Sarajevo school teacher during the siege
10. Ethnic map of the Republics of Croatia and of Bosnia and Herzegovina
11. UN protected areas crosshatched map
12. W140 Humanitarian relief
13. Air lift
14. Health monitor – 18th Jan 1992
15. Health monitor – 20th Nov 1992
16. Dagestan – no equipment but loving care
17. Third degree burns, Sarajevo
18. Dagestan willing hands but no equipment
19. A primitive artificial leg but Sarajevo willing hands
20. The basic elements for survival
21. Surgical oxygen – Sarajevo basement
22. My grandfather, Joseph Rennoldson's shipbuilding company built Lady Brassey
23. Dr Douglas McAlpine – Senior Neurologist, Middlesex Hospital Medical School

CHAPTER 1
The Social Lesion Defined

The word 'lesion' in the title of this book is borrowed from clinical science where it is used to denote structural change somewhere in the body caused by injury or disease. Much of our work as doctors is devoted to trying to discover where 'the lesion' responsible for a patient's symptoms is and what to do about it. Is a pain in the chest on exertion due to a lesion (narrowing) in a coronary artery supplying the heart muscle with blood or to something else? Likewise if someone complains that a foot drags on walking is the 'lesion' causing the weakness in one of the nerves supplying the leg or is it in the spinal cord or even the brain? Many of us who have been medical students have excruciating memories of embarrassment when at the patient's bedside our teachers tried unavailingly to coax us towards a logical approach to diagnosis along these lines.

But lesions can also have a sinister aspect. Sometimes like high blood pressure they may exist undisclosed for years before causing symptoms while in the meantime they gradually impair health by increasing the burden on the heart. As for others, (like a cold in the head or an upset stomach), will they get better without treatment or at the other extreme defy all our efforts as doctors and have a fatal outcome? Or, as is more often the case turns out to be somewhere in between? Quite recently, long after I had given up clinical practice, but with my experiences in Bosnia organising humanitarian relief fresh in mind, it occurred to me that a parallel to lesions within the human body may exist in society. This idea resonated with my childhood in Belfast where over the years tensions between Catholics and Protestants had led to a seemingly endless cycle of eruptions of civil disorder. Could 'social lesions' also have been at the heart of civil unrest which has beset so many other countries of the world – Indonesia, Rwanda-Burundi and Sri Lanka to mention but three since World War Two with Kosovo and Darfur as more recent examples.

I have a clear memory of the moment when this idea took definite shape in my mind. It was a Sunday in 1992 and I was in wartime Sarajevo as the World Health Organisation's (WHO) Special Representative in Former Yugoslavia. I had just emerged into the central square from one of the city's two cathedrals. My Nepalese driver and bodyguard were sitting smoking on top of the United Nations High Commission for Refugee's (UNHCR) Armoured Personnel Carrier (APC) which had just brought me the two kilometres from my office at the other end of 'sniper's alley'. As we walked down the steps my Bosnian doctor friend put his hand on my shoulder.

> *"Stop a minute!"* he said. *"From where we are standing you can see not only the other cathedral which is for people of the Serbian Orthodox faith"*, and he pointed, *"but also the Mosque and the Synagogue all within one hundred metres of each other".*

And almost in tears he went on;

> *"Can anything speak more eloquently for tolerance than that? In this city for centuries we lived together in peace and worshipped as we pleased: in Bosnia the religious wars of Europe never touched us".*

> *"And now in Sarajevo here we are besieged by the Serbs; with 250,000 people under bombardment and without electricity or gas while elsewhere in Bosnia the various groups are murdering each other! Will you please explain to me what has happened?"*

I had no answer.

A few weeks later once again in Sarajevo I was asked the same question but in a different context. This time I was trying to find out what was happening to elderly people. In the absence of both shops and public transport had they been able to brave the snipers and collect their UNCHR rations or were they starving? The man who stopped me to speak with him in the street on this occasion turned out to be a retired teacher. He was desperately thin and his daughter with whom he lived had already bartered most of their possessions for food and candles. But before he was prepared to discuss their plight or his dread of the coming winter there was something as a teacher he wanted urgently to tell me.

> *"For the last twenty years all our children here have been in mixed schools and we have taught them they have equal rights. Now the same children are killing each other! Why?"*

To use my analogy based on human disease, what had happened in Sarajevo and indeed through much of Yugoslavia was that hidden tensions within society – between Croats, Serbs and Muslims – which for many years had caused no apparent symptoms had now erupted into the psychological equivalent of a cancerous growth, the end point of which was genocide.

A Model of the Social Lesion

My ideas about communities where there is a social lesion are modelled in the diagram.

As an example I use the simplest case where there are two groups – the 'haves' and 'have nots' divided by race, religion or wealth or a combination of these.

Within such a community a sustained sense of tension exists between the groups, one of which sees itself as superior and in control, the other inferior and helpless. The group which considers itself in control (Group A) perceives a potential threat from Group B which leads to feelings of insecurity and fear for the future. The group without control feels frustrated and angry because it is excluded from economic opportunity and a right to express its cultural identity. A situation where the 'social lesion' is accompanied by differences in physical appearance such as skin colour or by religion seems to lead to sharper divisions than those expressed exclusively in terms of social position and wealth.

Social lesions may lie latent within a community for generations without any apparent detriment and only come to the surface as the result of misconceived activities of politicians or religious leaders. At this point the lesion is no longer latent but has entered a downward spiral where prejudice (Stage 1) leads to intimidation and segregation. Stage 2 involves sporadic or cyclical violence e.g. shop smashing, arson, looting and riots. In the final stage (Stage 3) government itself enters the arena either to keep the peace or alas sometimes the opposite by using police or the military to orchestrate such activities as 'ethnic cleansing', 'mass rape' and genocide.

All these situations in their various degrees have I believe recurred throughout history. In my own lifetime, quite apart from the 'troubles' in Ireland, and those during the break up of the Yugoslav Federation and in the Chechnyan region of Russia, in all three of which I have had personal experience, there have been genocidal disturbances in Rwanda and Burundi, in Sri Lanka and various other places most recently in Kosovo. The key point is that none of these conflicts came out of the blue. If we can learn from that there may be some hope for the future.

A Lesion

A structural change in a bodily part resulting from injury or disease.

A 'Social' Lesion

A sustained sense of tension between population groups one of which regards itself as superior to the other, which in turn feels inferior.

Group A - in Control

Perceives threats to its social and economic position from Group B. Feelings of insecurity and fear for the future.

Group B - without Control

Perceives exclusion from social and economic opportunity and suppression of its right to express its cultural identity. Feelings of frustration and anger against Group A.

STAGE 1

Personal and group discrimination.
Intimidation.
Fostering of prejudice.
Segregation.

STAGE 2

Sporadic or cyclical violence eg shop smashing, arson, looting, riots.

STAGE 3

Premeditated violence as an act of policy by police or armed forces.
Planned 'ethnic cleansing'.
Planned 'mass rape'.
Genocide.

A 'Social' Lesion
What to do about it?

Do

Recognise it.
Measure it.
Address it.

Don't

Ignore it.
Hope it will go away.
Reinforce it, or
Permit reinforcement
by media, public
speeches etc.

Figure 1. A model of the Social Lesion

To conclude my ideas on the social lesion I go back to an article I wrote in 1996[1]. While its title was *"Preventing Genocide"* this is relevant because as occurred in the Bosnian town of Srebrenica, the ultimate consequence of a social lesion maybe exactly that! For that very reason it is important that episodes of genocide and other degrees of civil disorder should not be allowed to pass without notice or international concern. To make the case I call in as an authority none other than Adolf Hitler himself.

In 1939 shortly before the German invasion of Poland, Hitler made a secret speech to his top military advisors in which he set out his plans for the settlement of Poland after the expected successful completion of the military campaign. I quote from his speech.

> *"Poland will be depopulated and settled with Germans"*,

he said. Just as Genghis Khan had, sent millions of women and children into death knowingly, and *"with a light heart"* he had ordered the SS to kill without mercy,

> *"women and children of Polish origin and language"*.

But in 1939 how would Germany escape condemnation for such a policy? That was the problem! There follows a key passage in the speech in which Hitler referred to a forgotten massacre in Turkey in the First World War when more than a million Armenian Christians were killed; I quote:

> *"After all who today is speaking of the destruction of the Armenians?"*

Perhaps we should invert Hitler's intention and turn his argument upside down. If it is possible for the world so soon to forget a horrendous genocide in which more than a million Armenians were killed perhaps action should be taken to ensure that such convenient oblivion does not occur again.

This leads me to suggest that episodes of civil unrest should not pass without record and analysis. The United Nations or a suitable non-political international agency of high standing such as the International Committee of the Red Cross should set up a centre which will become a global 'lighthouse' of information about civil unrest: it's objective being to discover, record, analyse and publicise episodes of civil unrest worldwide. The long term objective of this would be to promote better understanding of the dynamics of the 'social lesion' and to reduce its pernicious consequences. The issue of the Social Lesion and its consequences ought also to be discussed in schools and colleges as part of general education.

The hope which underlies this idea would be that such a centre would create a properly documented body of knowledge open to all. This would contribute to the development of policies which would reduce the risk of progression of social lesions to situations which in the past too often have led to violence and sometimes even genocide.

The illustration taken from a recent newspaper in England shows an episode of civil disorder in one of the islands in Indonesia. Something has happened which has led members of one ethnic group to try in desperation to leave. Seemingly at a moment's notice men, women and children are abandoning their homes and livelihoods without even the opportunity to collect their personal belongings, and fleeing for their lives to a country far away.

Yugoslavia: the land of the Southern Slavs

How was it that all of these events came about in Yugoslavia? An answer to this question requires a brief diversion into history. Yugoslavia, like Czechoslovakia was a country created in central Europe following the collapse of the Austro Hungarian Empire in 1919. During the Second World War Yugoslavia was invaded by Nazi Germany. The dominant group who ejected the Germans were the Partisans. This was led by Marshall Tito who although nominally a Communist and undoubtedly a despot had the vision and courage to keep his polyglot country consisting of Croats, Serbs, Slovenes, Bosnians, Montenegrins, Macedonians, Hungarians and Jews together until his death in 1980.

Tito is widely acclaimed for the resounding *"No"* on one occasion he gave to Stalin. This was in 1948 when the Russian dictator sought safe passage for the Red Army through his country to the Mediterranean – a move which if it had succeeded as well as destroying the independence of Yugoslavia would have had dire consequences for the Western democracies. Perhaps of equal importance but at the same time an ironic memorial to an atheist was Tito's much less well known policy of 'brotherhood and unity' which ran counter to racialism. In my travels in Yugoslavia I came upon a remarkable example of this. From Belgrade, Tito had provided money to build mosques in all the major towns of Bosnia, thus for the first time providing places of worship for the third largest population group in the country, and one that had generally been regarded by the Serbs and Croats as inferior. But even this, alas, was not enough to assuage the social tensions.

Towards the end of the Bosnian civil war and after I had left the Former Republic of Yugoslavia, two manifestations of the ultimate consequences of the 'social lesion' occurred, the second comparable to the atrocities committed in Hitler's Reich to sustain so-called racial purity. The first took place on 5th February 1994 when a mortar bomb deliberately aimed at the predominantly Muslim open market in the Markele sector of Sarajevo at a busy time killed 68 people many of them women and children and wounded many more. If that can be thought of as a possible accident, the next example on a much greater scale cannot have been accidental.

This was the cold-blooded massacre of several thousand young men and boys in the town of Srebrenica on 11th July 1995. Here was the 'social lesion' at its worst manifested in what is almost a defining example of genocide. General Milosevic of Serbia who had replaced Tito in Belgrade felt that a town a few miles from his border containing a significant pool of 'Moslem genes' was an intolerable threat to the future racial purity and security of his country. He therefore gave orders that all the male inhabitants under 60 years of age should be taken out and shot.

Two years previously, almost to the day, the RAF, as part of the United Nations Protective Force, (known as UNPROFOR) which flew supplies into Sarajevo and other so called 'protected areas' had invited me to visit Srebrenica in one of their helicopters. To my everlasting regret I declined because I did not think it was worthwhile as there was a time limit of six hours in the visit to enable the helicopter to get back before dark. When recently I asked a former colleague who had worked in FRY in humanitarian relief whether I had been at fault for not recognising the risk of a tragedy in Srebrenica and not opening a WHO office there as a preventative measure, he reminded me that a major decision such as that could only have been made by UNHCR who were in the political lead, not WHO. In his view, WHO's role was quite clearly limited to health. This is all very well but the fact remains that if I had had the wit to foresee what was likely to happen in Srebrenica and scraped together the resources to open a WHO office there I doubt whether anyone would have gainsaid me.

If I had gone would I have spotted that tragedy was inevitable? And if so would I have warned Britain's Prime Minister, John Major with whom in those days I had a close link? After all Srebrenica was an obvious target for genocide. As well as being a Muslim enclave close to the Serbian border, it was by this time conveniently packed with refugees of like religion from the neighbouring enclaves of Zepa and Gorazde.

The census of 1990, ethnic cleansing and mass rape
In 1990, a short time before I arrived in Yugoslavia, President Milosevic decided that there should be a census and that everyone within the Federation should be required to declare not only name, address, age etc, but – ominously - in addition to the usual information, their 'race'. I remember well the young local people who were employed in my office telling me that, after a generation of Tito's relaxed despotism since World War Two many of them had to consult their grandparents about race as they had no idea what to write. From this census coloured maps emerged-still available-showing for each town and district 'pie-charts' which displayed its racial profile-blue for Serb, red for Croat and green for Moslem. These later became the template for ethnic cleansing.

And what exactly was 'ethnic cleansing'? A town or village was said to have been 'cleansed' when one group (usually but not exclusively the Serbs) had succeeded in getting rid of the others. This might be achieved by forced eviction, the signing over of land under duress, by intimidation of all kinds, by partial or completely razing the villages or in the ultimate by massacre.

In addition, a spectre from the past, the technique of laying siege to towns emerged in Europe for the first time since the siege of Leningrad in 1941. Sarajevo, where the siege lasted more than three years was the best known but by no means the only town so affected. Other besieged towns such as the predominantly Moslem enclaves of Zepa, Gorazde and Srebrenica close to the Serbian border which I have already mentioned, although much smaller than Sarajevo, were in some ways less fortunate as they had no airfields and it was more difficult for the UN authorities to negotiate supplies for them with the besiegers.

Many of the Bosnian towns – like Sarajevo itself – are surrounded by hills. It was in such hills that the Serbs placed their artillery and by intermittent indiscriminate bombardments, sealing off access to food and interrupting the public water supply tried to force the people to leave.

When, as happened in the Moslem town of Jajce, the population could take no more, a road was opened to let the women, children and the elderly out to swell the numbers of dispossessed on the other side of the line. A worse fate was often reserved for men of military age. Raising the siege of this beautiful town had an unexpected consequence which, as I am an epidemiologist, was brought to my attention. The tracks of the people on their escape route to the coast became mysteriously peppered with cases of typhoid fever. I discovered that some years previously there had been an epidemic of typhoid in Jajce due to an infected water source which had never been properly remedied. Fortunately there were no deaths and the outbreak ceased without fatalities. Hopefully the relevant spring has since been dealt with by the local public health authorities.

During the period I was working in Former Yugoslavia ethnic cleansing had already led to the ejection of a huge number of people. UNHCR told me that there were about 2 million people in temporary residence in other people's homes or in refugee centres and that within the besieged enclaves a further million also depended upon humanitarian aid for food and medical supplies. On one occasion when I was in the predominantly Serbian town of Banja Luka evaluating the local hospital's needs for surgical supplies I heard that major 'cleansing' (i.e. massacre) of the minority groups was imminent. Fortunately I was able to get in touch with David Owen who with Cyrus Vance, his American partner in the 'Vance-Owen' agreement dropped everything to come at once and stabilise the situation.

Mass Rape

While I was working in Bosnia I heard rumours that young Moslem women were being held in custody in 'rape camps' to serve as involuntary prostitutes and a photograph was given to me as evidence. Probably because I took the word 'camp' too literally I was not able personally to confirm the existence of the so-called 'rape camps' on the spot. Quite recently I discovered that in fact the girls abused in this manner were more likely to have been detained in schools or community 'sports centres' than in 'camps'. While I was working there I did however come across a tragic case of rape with the offensive racial overtones which it is now clear was typical of what was happening in many places in Bosnia. My informant was a lady who was Director of the Red Cross in Slavonski Brod. The young Bosnian woman in question had been repeatedly raped by Serb soldiers and kept forcibly in custody until she was eight months pregnant and then released. She refused to see the baby – a lovely little boy fortunately unaware of these deplorable events – who I saw happily asleep in his cot and who I was told was about to be adopted.

Later in the war after I had left Yugoslavia a detailed first hand account of the experiences of twenty five young women in one of the 'rape camps' was published in the scientific literature[1].

As it corroborates what I had heard second-hand I reproduce verbatim an account of the experiences of one of a group of twenty five young women thus abused.

> *"Ms. C. was a 16 year old Moslem peasant girl from Bosnia. Together with her mother and 10 year old sister she was taken from her village to a detention camp. She is uncertain about the camp's location because they arrived there at night (in trucks with Yugoslav Federal Army insignia) and she never left the building where she was detained. There she shared a room with twelve other girls aged 12-30; all of them were raped almost every day by soldiers. After five months she escaped.*
>
> *...After her arrival in Zagreb Ms. C. was hospitalised with an advanced pregnancy... When asked about the baby which she was about to bear she answered curtly that she did not want to see it and would give it up for adoption. She experienced the fetus as foreign to her body and wanted to be rid of it".*

Five years after the end of the war a number of cases of 'sexual enslavement' were brought before the International Tribunal for Former Yugoslavia. In the predominantly Moslem town of Foca captured by the Serbs, Muslim women had been detained in the 'sports centre',

---

[1] Kozaric-Kovacic, D., et al. 1995 Amer J. Orthopsychiatr. 65 (3) pp428-433

motels and the primary school where they were subjected to sexual abuse of all kinds including rape and gang rape.[2]

Similar crimes are reported to have been committed also by Croat and Moslem men against Serb women although less frequently.[3]

These episodes of gang rape and sexual abuse perpetrated along ethnic lines in Former Yugoslavia during its recent wars seem to me to be the ultimate expression of the existence of a 'social lesion' as I have defined it. This is because they imply premeditated malice towards a generation yet unborn as well as causing grave psychological and physical injury to the women.

Targeting hospitals

Another deplorable consequence of the 'social lesion' in the Former Republic of Yugoslavia was the deliberate targeting of hospitals by artillery. How could we be sure the damage was deliberate? I will give three examples. In Vukovar in Croatia, the local hospital was bombarded at close range by tanks and rockets between September 1991 and January 1992. When I visited it in July 1992 the interior was still in an indescribable mess and clinical work was being conducted in the basement. In the medical library on the top floor and in the operating theatre I was shown the wires of hand held rockets which had been guided through the windows from a launcher a few hundred metres away.

---

[2] Bosnian Rape camp trial opens. 20/3/00 BBC News http://news.bbc.co.uk/i/li/worl…
    The indictment ("Foca") http://www..un.org/icty/glance/
     Case information shut 13/1/03. http/www.un.org/icty/glance
[3] Commission on human rights. 49th session. Agenda item Z7
Situation of human rights in the territory of Former Yugoslavia E/CN.4/1993/50. 10/2/93

In Breza, a town on the front line near Sarajevo the x-ray department, the pharmacy and the pathology laboratory had each received a direct hit by a mortar bomb two weeks before my visit. In Bihac, the large regional hospital which stands alone in its own grounds and could not possibly be mistaken for a military target received several direct hits, one of which killed twelve patients sitting at a table having lunch in a ward and wounded several others. My horror at this atrocity led me to approach Margaret Thatcher who at that time had just stepped down as Britain's Prime Minister to use her influence to stop this happening again. She responded immediately and thanks to her intervention the ICRC declared the hospital a protected area. But as has so often been the case elsewhere in human history, in Bosnia also heroism often matched the horrors, and the conduct of the medical and nursing professions was exemplary almost everywhere. Time and time again I visited hospitals which had been damaged by gunfire where emergency surgery was still being carried out, the staff continuing to work on the ground floor or in the basements, and morale was excellent. Winter brought with it the additional problem that very few areas in the hospitals could be heated, electricity was intermittent and in Sarajevo there was often hardly any water. On one occasion a colleague of mine in that city assisted at an emergency surgical operation being conducted in a theatre where the ambient temperature was at freezing point (0°). I do not know whether the patient survived.

On the shores of the Caspian Sea

Early in 1995 I found myself in Central Asia once again under the flag of WHO. There had been serious civil disturbances in the Chechnya area of the Russian Federation, tens of thousands of displaced persons were on the roads and rumours were circulating of outbreaks of cholera, plague and other infectious diseases. Once again Lynda Chalker, the

UK's Minister for Overseas Development sent for me. I remember the occasion well.

> *"This time let's see if we can leave something constructive behind when the disturbances are over", she said. And she went on with a twinkle; "By the way you will have the full support of the Russian Government, they appear to know you quite well".*

She was right on her final point. Although I could not claim to be a pal of Mr Kruschev or his henchmen I did at least have a more than passing acquaintance with Russia's representatives at the World Health Organisation. There was an amusing reason for this. At meetings of the World Health Assembly in Geneva which I attended for several years, the seating was arranged alphabetically by country – the UK delegation which I led therefore being seated adjacent to the USSR at the back of the hall. Due to our strategic location not only near the exits but the toilets and the bar, a certain conviviality developed between us. This was fostered by the fact that the stuffy members of the U.S. delegation (our neighbours on the other side for the same alphabetic reason) kept themselves very much to themselves.

So having once again accepted Lynda Chalker's invitation, over the next two years I was to pay a series of brief visits to the States of the Russian Federation which are situated at the foot of Caucasus mountains on the shores of the Caspian Sea – Dagestan, Ingushetia and Ossetia, and which in those days were not usually open to foreigners.

And were the disturbances in the Caspian region also due to a "sustained sense of tension between two population groups" – in other words a "social lesion"? They turned out to be no exception! In this case the two groups involved were the Russian colonists (historically

Orthodox Christians) who regarded themselves as superior and the indigenous Muslim population who saw themselves as the conquered. Over the centuries, as might be expected, the Russians had secured most of the positions of power as well as social and linguistic dominance. In Moscow the prevailing attitude of the Russians towards the indigenous people had been given away when I was being briefed by a senior official in their Ministry of Health.

Referring to a recent grant, the Russian Government had received from the International Committee of the Red Cross, he commented in wonderment,

> *"Do you know that the ICRC actually goes so far as to insist that we must use their money to help the Chechens on equal terms to us Russians?"*

To which I added, untactfully but with a smile *"and so will WHO!"*

I enter a time warp

But a thousand miles from Moscow as my kind hosts escorted me through the clinics and hospitals in Makhachkala, Vladikavkaz and Nasran, it became clear that there must be factors other than the 'social lesion' to explain the catastrophic situation which emerged. In a country with a nuclear capability which had recently put men on the moon, health care had collapsed and unlike the situation in the Former Republic of Yugoslavia was now on a par with services in the poorest countries of the world. Thus there had been no immunisation in many parts of the region for three years; the 'cold chain' which keeps vaccines and various medicines chilled in transit between manufacturer and patient had broken down and the hospitals had little or no equipment in the laboratories or wards. Worst of all there was an epidemic of tuberculosis which was being treated with outdated and dangerous methods. These risked the creation of new strains of the bacterium which would not only defy all available remedies but would almost certainly spread elsewhere.

In my travels I found a situation full of contrasts and surprises: the shore of the Caspian Sea on a breezy day where, on a beach lapped by filthy water and littered with rubbish, at the same time fitness fiends were jogging and doing their exercises; a hospital for handicapped children where the kids were cared for devotedly by nurses - no hint of an 'euthanasia' policy there – but had been abandoned by their families; and a centre for displaced persons where the women living there took their shoes off on entering and worked hard with brooms and dust pans to keep the hostel spotlessly clean. However, the same hostel had no clean drinking water and the latrines stank. As for WHO, how could we contribute to help this situation? Generous shipments of our standard kits for mothers and babies; for surgical operations; for anaesthetics and for mental hospitals, which I had ordered had all arrived – but in the sense of Lynda Chalker's hopes – their benefit was temporary. In the longer term WHO's gift of a range of laboratory equipment including some up to date microscopes together with information about modern methods of treating tuberculosis (the WHO protocol) will have been even more helpful.

As for myself, I take away two vivid recollections of my trips to the Russian Federation, one tragic, one happy. Even now, years later I am sometimes haunted when wakeful by the expression on the face of a small boy no more than six years old sitting legs crossed on the edge of a street in Moscow. He had lost one eye and he was totally alone, begging, playing a miniature violin with his cap upturned on the pavement in front of him and he told me he had no living relations. A soup kitchen provided one basic meal of bread and soup when he felt strong enough to walk to the distribution point. No other social support apparently in the capital of a Communist country.

But then I think of the expressions on the faces of the two heroic white-coated ladies in the laboratory in the hospital in Vladikavkaz a thousand miles away, when they told me that the bacteriological kits and the modern microscope from WHO had transformed their practice and were far and away the most useful help they had ever received.[4]

As far as the Chechnyan region itself is concerned I heard later that the war gave way to anarchy, a Finnish colleague who had been advising on the reconstruction of damaged buildings had been murdered and it had become too dangerous for foreigners to visit. Russians living locally whose houses had been destroyed had received compensation sufficient to enable them to rebuild anywhere in the Federation; but Chechens in similar plight had been given just enough money to rebuild on the spot.

Would this manifestation of the 'social lesion' increase or reduce the risk of future discord and conflict I wondered? I cannot say. But I feel certain that in the Caucasus region of Russia the 'social lesion' survived the Chechnyan war.

---

[4] Their microscopes which we replaced with a modern binocular model seemed to be an exact replica of those provided at Oxford for each medical student in the class, where almost fifty years previously I had been taught the elements of bacteriology

CHAPTER 2
Health, Humanitarian Relief, and Survival in Former Yugoslavia

By the time I arrived in the 'Former Republic of Yugoslavia' on 12th July 1992 as WHO's Special Representative, the United Nations had for good or ill made three crucial political decisions which would set the scene for my work in the coming months. The first was that it would not go to war with Serbia, the initial aggressor. Instead it would put pressure on that country to mend its ways by punitive sanctions barring it to international trade and restricting its imports to a very short list of essentials. The UN's second decision was that in the meantime it would protect and support refugees and displaced persons throughout the country whether Serb, Croat or Muslim - including three hundred thousand people billeted in hotels, schools and private houses on the Dalmatian coast. Thirdly, and this turned out to have been wildly optimistic, instead of raising the siege of Sarajevo immediately by armed force, the UN would supply its population of circa 250,000 men, women and children by 'airlift' for what it hoped would be a few weeks – as had been successful in the siege of West Berlin in the 'cold war' of the 1950's. In the same way, the smaller Muslim enclaves of Gorazde, Zepa and Srebrenica were to be provisioned by UNCHR land convoys protected by escorts of UNPROFOR armoured cars. At the time these decisions were made no one could have predicted that the war and the virtual imprisonment of all these people was to continue for more than three years.

In Geneva where I was briefed for my task, it was not surprising bearing in mind the way the international community had tied their hands, that I found the headquarters officials of UNHCR and WHO in a state of unmitigated frustration and gloom. My most vivid recollection is of my briefing about the care of refugees and displaced persons from a man whose experience had ranged across almost all the continents and disturbances since the end of World War Two.

"Shelter, warmth and clean water on the same day as they arrive are your top priorities", he said. "They are a must!" "As for food, they can do without that for a day or two at a pinch, and UNHCR will be there with their rations well before the end of the week!" "But what about their health", I asked, "they may have been on the road for weeks?" "Setting aside the babies who are a special case, that will become clear soon enough", he said. "Don't go running around with a stethoscope and a patella hammer, just count the people and count the deaths. If you have 1 death per 1000 per week, you have a serious problem, and if you have more, a potential disaster". What's more a sample of the dying and dead give you a lead as to what are the prevalent diseases.

Casting my mind back to my student days when I was taught that the death rate in England was approximately 3 per 1000 per annum, I got the message.

My Task

My task, bearing in mind that I was already past the usual age of retirement, was challenging to say the least. In a mountainous, polyglot war stricken country, while observing strict neutrality at all times, I was to feed back information urgently to Geneva not only about the health of the people in the refugee camps but also about those in the UN Protected Areas and above all, within the besieged cities and towns. Unfortunately as a few days earlier in an unprecedented tragedy the Chief Delegate of the ICRC (International Committee of the Red Cross) had been killed on the road to Sarajevo when a 'cleared' convoy he was leading had been bombarded by mortars, I was enjoined to 'take good care of myself'. As for money, WHO had provided enough for a small office in Zagreb, together with a secretary and a Nissan 'Patrol' car complete with driver. Anything else I might need to cope with the catastrophic situation was to be raised by my own efforts from what the bureaucrats cheerfully called 'as yet unidentified sources.' My boss, in theory, at any rate, was WHO's Regional Director for Europe in faraway Copenhagen. But as the last time WHO had been involved in humanitarian relief was forty years previously in the Congo there was little practical experience in that quarter on which to draw.

As my train rumbled into Zagreb station after a 30 hour journey – no civilian air flights being available because of the war – I was tired, jaded and indeed dejected. Where in the world would I raise money on the scale to make a difference? But as I stepped down from the train two cheerful people were there to greet me – one an attractive young woman called Sanja Viscovic, who spoke perfect English with a slight American accent, the other also smiling but with a good deal less English - Branko Pelko – who was to be my driver. His taxi would be my official car. My gloom began to lift. At least we could make a start.

An office had already been organised – albeit with a box turned upside down as my desk and a 'local calls only' telephone – and I had been booked in at a comfortable hotel in town. But most important of all was the atmosphere of invincible optimism. We were on our way! Without the unfailing support and encouragement of these two individuals during the year that followed I would have accomplished nothing. The following excerpts from my diary describe my first impressions and a very steep learning curve.

13th July

Today I met the boss (Special Representative) of the UN humanitarian efforts here – a charismatic Spaniard called José Maria Menduluce: extremely anxious about the immediate fate of 1.6 million displaced persons, on the road or in makeshift accommodation. He was also concerned about the besieged cities of which Sarajevo is the largest and crowded with refugees.

Then Melhuish, ex-UK Ambassador to Thailand who is Head of the EU Mission here. He has 140 monitors who are trying to enforce the 'ceasefire' between Croatia and Serbia and asks could these monitors also report to me on health in these areas?

It was almost immediately after my arrival that I heard the unpleasant term 'ethnic cleansing' for the first time and learned that genocide was being practised by all sides.

When my Croatian hosts showed me a book which claimed that all atrocities were Serbian, instead of accepting it with a smile and without comment, I stupidly gave them a lecture on my neutrality. This ill timed and facile display of tactlessness went down badly and was to lead, I later discovered, to a stream of 'black' propaganda about my 'licentious and immoral activities' being sent from Zagreb to my boss the Regional Director in Copenhagen.

20ᵗʰ July

A mortar attack on the airport at Sarajevo has interrupted the airlift making my first trip there more difficult to arrange. Iset Aganovic, a senior Moslem doctor has called in to see me. He tells of a direct hit on a shelter in the small town of Gorazde which killed or wounded more than one hundred people and of a young colleague who has undertaken 6 amputations without anaesthetics in the last few days. He tells me what he regards as the four most urgent priorities which take precedence over all others:

External fixation equipment – (to stabilise shattered limbs while the damage heals)
   Anaesthetics
   Antibiotics
   Analgesics

As light relief to this grim catalogue he tells me that some ass in Geneva presumably imagining that Sarajevo is in the tropics, has sent a consignment of 'kits' to combat malaria, amoebic dysentery and plague. This last fiasco took us months to live down and led to WHO being branded as a bunch of amateurs. In addition to these totally inappropriate ingredients within the UN's supplies there was also a serious omission. The food did not contain micronutrients. To my astonishment I discovered that UNCHR's standard ration for global use had <u>no</u> <u>vitamins,</u> indeed it transpired that recently a famine struck population in East Africa had actually developed scurvy due to the absence of Vitamin C (ascorbic acid) in the relief rations provided by the United Nations. In the weeks that followed I arranged that vitamins in suitable quantities should be delivered to every household in Sarajevo. For the rest of the siege Vitamin C became a talisman for health and survival, with psychological benefits far beyond anything that could realistically have been expected and overnight I had made 10,000.00 new friends.

21st July

Despite being here for only one week, two brothers who are doctors in a small Bosnian town have heard of my existence and have come to seek help. Their hospital which is under fire from tanks and other heavy weapons has two people to a bed and others sleeping on the floor. It has no anaesthetics and very few antibiotics and painkillers.

Unfortunately I have just sent all the supplies here to Sarajevo on the airlift but I swear I will get help to them somehow within the coming weeks.

The Gorazde Convoy

During the next nine months, having been too young to serve in WW2, I was to experience for the first time the excitement, the special sense of team work and the heightened awareness which comes with working at high risk for a good cause. But as the intensity of local nationalism was such that it was out of the question for Sanja or Branko to cross the border out of Croatia, it was obvious I would need additional locally staffed offices in other parts of Former Yugoslavia - at least in Sarajevo and in Belgrade and probably elsewhere. But where on earth was the money to come from? I need not have worried! Events would soon follow which solved our financial problems for the rest of the war. When I left for home in April 1993, in addition to our headquarters in Zagreb, there were offices in Belgrade, Split and Sköpje, as well as in Sarajevo and we had received donations of more than $1 million US dollars in cash and several times as much in kind.

> **21st July 1992 (cont.)**
>
> *"I have had a call today from UNHCR's lead man in Sarajevo, Tony Land to try and sort out the drug and equipment distribution problems there. Of course I agreed. Apparently the equipment etc. does not get to the wards, and appears to be being stock piled somewhere or stolen".*

> **22nd July 1992**
>
> *"Sitting in a Hercules aircraft flown by the Italian Air force bound for Sarajevo as part of the UN's humanitarian airlift. The flight takes*

one hour and fifteen minutes and is roundabout via Split to avoid Serb anti-aircraft missiles. My seat is one of two rigged sideways against the shell of the aircraft facing inwards. The fuselage contains pallets of humanitarian supplies plus one oxygen concentrator. 'Concentrators' draw the oxygen from the air using ordinary mains electric current and are for personal delivery by me to one of the operating theatres of the main (Kosovo) hospital in Sarajevo[5]. I had intended to take three but in the light of recent events (I had met two doctors from a remote hospital in Bosnia who were having to operate without anaesthetics) I am retaining two of them. I have just been presented with a pair of earplugs and a steaming mug of cocoa. Two of the crew are reclining on the top of the pallets having scrambled past me".

Shortly afterwards this same plane was shot down in mysterious circumstances by a missile while on a similar trip to Sarajevo.[6] Many years later I was told that unknown to those in the UNHCR plane, there was a Serb fighter plane on its tail. A ground to air missile was fired at the fighter by Croatian forces and unfortunately hit the supply plane. All aboard including the steward who had presented me with earplugs and a mug of cocoa were killed. This tragedy had a profound effect on me. It not only removed any last trace of misunderstanding I had about the merciless nature of the Yugoslavian war but rendered my personal determination to help implacable.

---

[5] The oxygen essential for anaesthetics usually comes from specially designed high pressure cylinders which in the circumstances of civil war UNCHR refused to transport by air because they are dangerously flammable.

[6] At the end of the war it transpired this had been an accident. The UN plane was being shadowed by a Serb fighter, at which the Croats aimed a rocket. This missed its target but hit the Hercules which crashed in flames.

23rd July 1992

"On arrival in Sarajevo I found the first UNHCR convoy of humanitarian aid for Gorazde was about to leave. (Goradze was a remote Bosnian town with a Moslem majority in the midst of a Serbian contested area.) Commandeering some medicines available in a UN shipment at the airport and a WHO flag I cadged a lift in a Nissan Patrol Jeep with Fabricio Hochschild, a young Chilean who is leading the convoy and his interpreter. To reach Gorazde, we first of all had to take a circuitous route through the forest to avoid areas where there was fighting and then negotiate safe passage across the front line. The convoy consists of one armoured personnel carrier (APC) manned by UN troops in the lead and another at the rear, and with two twenty ton trucks driven by Swedish volunteers laden with supplies and our jeep in the middle. Our Armoured Personnel Carriers gave some protection from snipers provided one kept one's head down, but were not strong enough to help if we were to drive accidentally over a landmine. Fortunately by luck and common sense we survived.

As we passed out of Sarajevo across the airport there was some uncomfortably close sniper fire – whiz - ting, whiz – ting – which seemed to be directed at us – my first life experience of being fired at with live ammunition.[7] Fabricio and his interpreter did not budge so neither did I. Such is the force of example. By round about ways through road blocks and parleys we slowly wound our way through Bosnia. But 15km from Gorazde disaster struck as the APC immediately in front of us ran over a mine with a huge explosion and

---

[7] Later, after our safe return to Sarajevo when I was debriefing to General MacKenzie the Canadian Officer in command of UNHCR, he told me this had been a deliberate attempt by the Serbs to stop the convoy by assassinating Fabricio and me.

flash of light. My driver, my interpreter and I were perhaps 15 metres behind but fortunately our windscreen was not shattered. The place was a classic ambush position: a narrow dirt road in the forest on a steep upward incline with hairpin bends. Immediately after the explosion all hell broke loose with close firing from both sides of the road. All of us not in armoured vehicles dived for the ditch. Fortunately no one was hurt but after spending a chilly night in the open, the decision came that we should turn back".

On this occasion Gorazde was not relieved nor was it by the second convoy some weeks later. A third was successful. But that was not the end of the story. A surprising turn of events gave the first convoy to Gorazde, a significance for the future that none of us could have predicted. As I emerged from the ditch brushing my coat clean of leaves and twigs I encountered some totally unexpected visitors. Unknown to us, a German TV crew equipped with all their gear had been following the convoy through the forest. They soon spotted me as someone who through my work on HIV and AIDS as the UK's Chief Medical Officer had an international media profile. The interview I gave, leaning against the damaged APC and with the forest as background received global coverage and helped to alert the world to the reality of what was happening in Bosnia. It also showed WHO had decided on a hands-on approach. Over the succeeding months money poured in for medical equipment and supplies and WHO's overdraft vanished like mid-summer snow.

While we passed an extremely chilly night, without further ado, a relief convoy with heavy lifting equipment was setting out from UN headquarters to 'evacuate' us. This eventually arrived early the following evening, and having done a quick turnaround we all left in a single cavalcade as dusk was falling. Although this meant we would have to traverse the war zone in the dark it had the advantage that no new mines were likely to have been laid. Our cavalcade, which drove with lights on through at least one area where fighting was actually taking place, was as follows:

APC;

Communications truck;

Supplies truck (UNHCR);

APC;

Nissan Jeep with Fabricio, interpreter and myself;

Mobile crane;

Mobile crane with heavy vehicle transporter (damaged APC aboard);

Rear APC.

This extraordinary collection of vehicles with blazing headlights seemed to have a hypnotic effect on the combatants. In Rogatica, both sides ceased firing at each other as we drove down the main street only to recommence immediately we had passed.

The remainder of the night was spent parked in a safe area. Fabricio, Una, my interpreter and I dined off French military rations (widely acknowledge to be the best) cooked in the open on a solid fuel heater washed down with the contents of a bottle of Slibovic (local plum brandy) bought from a nearby farmer for $5 US dollars. It was a good moment in an extraordinary, disappointing and at times terrifying two days. Next time I decided we would travel with APC's only and no 'safe' vehicles – one of the APC's being packed with medicines and other supplies.

The worst moment had been lying in a ditch just outside Gorazde hearing the 'boom, boom, boom' of Serbian artillery shells falling at the rate of about two per minute on that small town. Next day, the fact that the conditions in the town were desperate was gleefully confirmed to me by a complacent Serbian colonel in command of the besiegers at the top of the hill who then promptly left for a two hour lunch break with his sister. Little did he realise how soon he would get his own come-uppance!

The two nights in the open also taught me something about the climate here. In a hot spell in July, by midnight it was uncomfortably chilly. The message I took away from this experience was that it would be calamitous if by Christmas we had failed to get the tens of thousands of refugees who were sleeping in tents or in the open in Bosnia under cover.

The mules have arrived

But the first Gorazde convoy had another sequel which as it turned out was good for morale. It gave us a cloak and dagger dare devil image which far from doing harm gave our operations a certain cachet. Having wearily driven our carefully packed medicines and equipment back to Sarajevo that was not the end of this story.

Four seemingly endless weeks later my office in Zagreb received a cryptic message. "The mules have arrived." That evening I went to bed with the satisfaction that thanks to one of the most ancient modes of transport employed by the human race – the mule - the two hundred kg of medicines which we had packed with such care were now safely in the hospital in Gorazde, having arrived by a roundabout route through the forest.

A massacre of pigs

But even that was not the end of Gorazde's story. By the end of September, the war had moved on and Gorazde was back in the hands of its Moslem majority. Against a background of burnt and looted Serb houses and corpses littering the streets, my colleague Larry Hollingsworth leading the next UNCHR convoy found that a massacre of pigs (a bizarre aspect of ethnic cleansing) had taken place. Pigs of course, although the source of various delicacies to Serbs are 'unclean' to Moslems. As the first UNCHR convoy to relieve Gorazde entered the town, the lead APC collided with a smart BMW. This, as might be expected was a write-off although none of its occupants (all of whom were drunk) was hurt.

"What was the appropriate administrative procedure?" Larry wondered.

"Exchange of insurance company particulars hardly seemed appropriate."

Fortunately it turned out that the car had just been stolen as booty of war from a burnt and deserted Serb house.

New responsibilities

Whether we liked it or not, the Gorazde convoy gave us a profile which changed our world forever and so the following months were dominated by a frenetic jumble of cries for help from all over Former Yugoslavia. The situation was further complicated when my friends in Zagreb began to realise that as WHO's Special Representative, I was bound by its charter to help the sick, wounded and homeless on all sides of the conflict regardless of whether they were Croats, Serbs or Bosnians, aggressors or victims of aggression. Many years later I learned that my strict observance of the UN policy of 'neutrality', unacceptable as it was to Croats, had led to a stream of 'black' propaganda about my activities reaching WHO's Regional Director in Copenhagen. This claimed that I was spending my time on drink and debauchery! The same concern – a determination that we should not be allowed 'to help the other side' had almost certainly been behind the sniping directed at Fabricio and myself as the convoy crossed Sarajevo Airport on the way to Gorazde.[8]

In the meantime, in my office in Zagreb - fortunately blissfully unaware of the slanderous news about me reaching Copenhagen - I decided on three elemental steps. I must cross the political 'line' and visit the capital of Serbia, Belgrade as soon as possible. I must expand rapidly and open the offices near points of need throughout the whole of the Former Republic of Yugoslavia, and I must find a way to package the enormous stock of medicines, dressings and bandages we were accumulating so that they could be easily available for use in the field. Last but not least, WHO must provide us with a proper administrative and financial structure to support what was rapidly becoming a large organisation.

Belgrade in wartime

In July 1992, Belgrade was grim. It showed what can happen to the capital of a small country if the rest of the world as represented by the United Nations 'sends it to Coventry' and applies sanctions.

As I land in UNPROFOR's six seater light aircraft the airport is closed and deserted. In my huge seemingly moribund hotel there are few guests and neither newspapers nor post – three week old copies of the New York Herald Tribune changing hands for $20 USD. The electric lights flicker dimly and the food although plentiful seemed tasteless – is even salt in short supply?

---

[8] UNCHR/WHO HQ. I slept there on numerous occasions during my visits to Sarajevo

Against this background, it is hardly surprising that Serbia is having difficulty coping with the influx of displaced persons and wounded from other parts of Former Yugoslavia. Nor that in the hospitals there are serious shortages of drugs and equipment with some categories already exhausted. Whatever their political views may be, the doctors and nurses I meet are devastated by their inability to cope with the stream of casualties arriving at their hospitals and WHO must help all sides in the conflict. My reaction is that Belgrade urgently needs a branch office of WHO and that it should have a share of the first delivery of medicines we receive.

The combination of good will and helpless incapacity which I encountered in Belgrade at that time was symbolised by a detail in the way the visit ended. I was invited to join my hosts who spoke perfect English, for dinner at an internationally renowned fish restaurant on the banks of the Danube. But in the absence of insecticides due to sanctions, clouds of hungry mosquitoes brought the meal to an abrupt conclusion at the end of the first course.

Back in Sarajevo

1st Sept 92[9]

Back in Sarajevo to which I was to make a total of eight brief visits over the following months – ostensibly to find two qualified observers locally ('focal points') in the jargon – to keep me in touch about local health, but also to make my own personal analysis.

But the general scene bears recording. At the airport, having been safely deposited by the Italian Hercules team of the airlift,

---

[9] The final flight of the UN airlift supplying the population of Sarajevo with food and other essentials was on 9 Jan 1996. Although the siege of that city having lasted almost three and a half years moral in the city did not collapse and the majority of the population survived.

increasingly tense as we made our approach – it was obvious that the security situation was more threatening. The PTT (Post-Telecommunications) building is now properly sandbagged by British Army sappers and the general security including barbed wire, and basement entry only is as it should have been months ago. Yet the international public servants of the UN (military and civil) who live in the PTT still do not have the least bit of entertainment (in the age of videos) or a choice of menu. No fruit has been seen in the canteen for months.

The fact that in addition to the civil war there is a direct threat to the UN itself is now obvious. Recently an APC flying the UN flag was attacked with a delayed action rocket. Unfortunately as one of the doors was open, one relief worker was killed and two others wounded.

And yet when I visited the local hospitals, although the old Jugoslav National Army Hospital has but one of its nine floors operative, with patients nursed away from the windows in the corridors to protect them from snipers, I found high morale everywhere. Fortunately the pre-war system of Health Clinics in almost every major street means that comparatively few people have to risk walking to hospital for care. The extraordinary spirit within the city is perhaps best exemplified by the blood bank which is still well stocked, with no shortage of donors who brave the snipers by walking to donation points from all over the city. The queues for bread at the bakery and for drinking water at the brewery are restrained and orderly. But autumn has not yet begun. In the bitter winter which occurs in this part of Europe – without power to heat the high rise blocks, no water to wash or flush toilets, and limited food rations what will happen to them then? I dread to think!

But most pitiable was the situation in the mental hospital. "How do you manage to care for acutely confused and disoriented patients at

*night without lights, let alone heating?" I asked. There was a long
pause: "Even some candles would be very helpful" came the answer.*

Six months later I found the situation in the mental hospital had
become critical. I was so shocked and horrified about a plan to
discharge a large number of seriously disturbed patients onto the streets
of the besieged city without any arrangements for their care or
protection that in a desperate effort to dissuade those in charge I visited
the Institute three times within a few days and on the third brought
Pieter Nielson UNHCR's Protection Officer with me. This stemmed the
crisis. Later at my request, WHO posted a distinguished and
courageous academic psychiatrist from India to Sarajevo to support the
local team and things improved for the remainder of the war.

Back in Zagreb, I was invited to go on TV and Radio including pieces
for the *Today* programme and BBC Breakfast TV. Money and staff on a
short term basis had begun to arrive, but in spite of the obvious need to
have offices in Sarajevo and Split, I still lacked even the minimum
financial assurances from WHO to enable me to plan for more than a
month at a time. After a sleepless night I made a crucial decision. In
retrospect it proved to have been the turning point which determined
the successful future of the WHO Humanitarian Relief project once and
for all. I decided to damn the lack of resources and seek urgent
professional advice in three fields – nutrition, winter protection and
pharmaceuticals regardless! From that day, a few weeks later when
these experts had arrived we never looked back. It seemed almost as if
somehow I had called the authorities' bluff and created a situation
which had shamed them into action and kits of clothing and medicines
arrived in abundance.

The shortage of medical supplies

When I arrived in Yugoslavia in July 1992, I quickly realised that quite contrary to my expectations, the pre-war standard of health care services was fully comparable to that in Britain and at least as expensive. There were 'ambulantes' – walk in clinics – easily accessible everywhere and in the hospitals there were specialists in all the familiar subjects – internal medicine, surgery, obstetrics, radiotherapy and so on working to a high standard, the majority of whom had done part of their training abroad. And yet, although almost everywhere the doctors and nurses had stayed at their posts, everything they needed be it medicines, anaesthetics, dressings, diagnostic equipment or artificial limbs was now in very short supply.

Our first attempt to solve the problem failed miserably. This was to ask the UK's Overseas Development Administration to send the range and quantity of medicines which would be needed for a moderately sized English town for a three month period. While this was fine for the purpose it was intended in Britain, namely for delivery to a wholesale pharmacy, in the conditions of a civil war where few if any pharmacies were open, the arrival of a Hercules aircraft laden with some hundreds of different packages labelled 'anaesthetics, analgesics, antibiotics', etc left us with an impossible logistical problem. It became obvious that we needed a different system and the services of a professional pharmacist.

What emerged was the 'kit' concept. This proved a great success and WHO continues to use and adapt it to deal with the various humanitarian relief crises which erupt across the world. The idea is to provide standard packages of essential medical supplies according to the needs of a defined population for a set period of time. These 'kits', are intended to deal with common illnesses and eventualities and contain large quantities of selected essential medicines rather than smaller amounts of a wider range of material.

By the time I left FRY in August 1993 our Director of Pharmacy, Dr Gilles Forté, had designed a total of no fewer than seventeen different kits covering every aspect of clinical practice, all of which have now stood the test of time and turned out to be much more useful in the field than a wide range of separately packaged medicines. In addition to covering the needs of primary healthcare, these emergency kits have also catered for reproductive health, chronic diseases and so on. Other kits are aimed to deal with the major communicable diseases such as pneumonia, tuberculosis and diarrhoea. Diagnostic kits were also developed to support hospital laboratories and surgical kits each provided materials for a specified number of elective or emergency operations. All were packaged in a way which would make handling locally as simple as possible e.g. for the general medical needs of a population of 1,000 people for three months; or for one hundred surgical operations, or obstetric deliveries or to meet the needs of a mental hospital with 100 patients for six months.

By the end of 1995, almost 64,000 kits including a variety of artificial limbs had been distributed by WHO with a total value of $24m and amounting to almost 2,000 tonnes. A recent post war evaluation concluded that despite some shortcomings 'the overall programme had been highly successful'. Behind this extraordinary story without which the clinical services in FRY would have collapsed, due credit should be given not only to the skill of the pharmacists who designed the 'kits' under the leadership of our Director of Pharmacy, Dr Gilles Forté, but also the courage of those who in conditions where the 'Red Cross' or 'Red Crescent' insignia were not always treated with respect, risked their lives crossing front lines and passing through war zones to distribute them.

One more river to cross

But there was a final problem to be solved in the area of medical supplies. How would we satisfy the need for surgical oxygen in the main operating theatres of the Kosovo Hospital in Sarajevo which were working day and night on military and civilian casualties and where it had turned out our simple 'concentrators' were insufficient to meet the need.

Once again ingenuity, the 'cloak and dagger' approach helped on this occasion by a generous benefaction from the Soros Foundation (Open Society Institute) in the USA solved the problem on this occasion. The parts of a large machine which together weighed nearly a ton were smuggled into Sarajevo from Britain and assembled under cover of darkness in the basement of the Hospital – a well kept secret to frustrate sabotage. There, for all I know, it remains today. Working on a diesel motor this machine extracted oxygen from the air and provided an ample supply even for lengthy and complicated procedures in overworked theatres for the rest of the war.

Siege, Starvation and Frostbite

Within a few weeks of my arrival in FRY in the autumn of 1992, I realised that for the first time in its 40 year history WHO had been asked to take responsibility for the health of a large civilian population in a besieged city. While it was for others to decide whether the siege should be raised by military means, as many of us on the spot felt strongly that was the appropriate action, our duty in the meantime was to work out what the essentials for the population's survival were and to do our best to ensure these were provided. The UN had taken the political decision not to go to war with the Serbian government but instead to support the population of Sarajevo by supplying it by air until a peace settlement was reached.

As I have already mentioned, by the time I took up my post in July 1992, the 'airlift' as it was called, was in full operation and Sarajevo was being supplied with food by military aircraft from Britain, France and Italy. While there was no doubt about the courage of the aircrew who often ran the gauntlet more than once a day knowing that any moment they might be fired on by Serb anti-aircraft batteries, at that time the appropriateness of their cargo in nutritional terms was open to question, as the cargo was composed exclusively of flour, rice and beans and in any case these staple foods were of little use without cooking fuel! Fortunately by coincidence, I had recently given a lecture[10] at Aberdeen's world famous 'Rowett Institute' on the government's role in nutrition, so I knew where exactly to turn for help.

> ### 5th September
>
> *Aileen Robertson, our nutritionist from the Rowett is already making an immense contribution to our work here. She has spotted immediately that the World Food Programme's rations unloaded from the Sarajevo 'airlift'* <u>*contain no micronutrients.*</u>
>
> *As they are virtually the only food available in Sarajevo we are therefore sailing straight towards outbreaks of scurvy, pellagra etc. My disbelief and incredulity that the UN's global programme to combat starvation fails to take into account principles about vitamins taught in schools throughout the world is beyond bounds. Aileen has pointed me to a recent article in the British Medical Journal which*

---

[10] The title was *Food, Nutrition and Government.*

described a serious outbreak in an East African country which caused many deaths while it was dependent on the UN for its supply of food.

Our remedy as well as being extremely popular was simple, effective and cheap. We commissioned a small factory in Sarajevo to make millions of tablets of ascorbic acid (vitamin C) and arranged for a consignment of all the other vitamins to be imported by air. Willing volunteers then braved the snipers to distribute the vitamins throughout the city, door to door. No doubt partly for psychological reasons everyone felt much better and WHO's popularity surged.

Three days ago 14 people queuing for water in Sarajevo were killed by a mortar bomb. One little boy aged 3 was left without parents.

Low Temperature Survival

In September, the days were getting shorter and even in Zagreb where I had opened my head office the evenings were cooler. Yet here we were virtually at sea-level while in Sarajevo in Bosnia some one hundred miles away the altitude of the city was 3000 feet above sea level – equivalent in Britain to the top of Snowdon! After all, some years previously, because Sarajevo could be relied on to have two or three metres of snow and a temperature of -5-10°C at night in January, the city had been chosen to host the Winter Olympic Games. Without access to coal or reliable supplies of either electricity or gas what would become of Sarajevo's two hundred and fifty thousand men, women and children when winter set in?

10th September

Reflections on Yugoslavia as I walk from my office to my favourite fish restaurant in decorous and almost smart Zagreb. The parks are full of lovers with nothing more exciting happening than the girl sitting on the lad's knee – no whores or thieves work here. The streets are cleaned daily and there is a marvellous cheap public transport system. Barely 100kms away in Banja Luka every type of ghastly atrocity has been committed and the Director of the Hospital brags to me that he has stated publicly that he does not think it is an appropriate place for little Moslems to be born; worse that the progeny of mixed Serb/Moslem marriages should be made into soap. How is it that such people have been boasting about murders and torture in public without any fear of being called to account?

Yesterday the priority was to send a message about the Sarajevo position to John Major (he had recently succeeded Margaret Thatcher as Prime Minister) who has asked me to keep him in touch. This I have done and he now knows that without the opening of the Mostar route, Sarajevo will starve before the end of the winter if they have not previously frozen to death. John Major gave unstinted moral support throughout my time in former Yugoslavia.

A Jewish doctor and his wife who have recently escaped from Sarajevo have given me a further first hand account of the imminent catastrophe. In addition to starvation, the lack of soap, toilet paper, disinfectants, insecticides, tampons etc (none of which are included in UNHCR's aid parcels) will they believe lead to outbreaks of infectious diseases.

12th September

I have reached a point of crisis. I am not prepared to sit here in Zagreb in a small office without funds and helpless while a humanitarian crisis develops in Bosnia. I will appeal to my friends in the European Commission and put my case personally at the meeting of WHO's Regional Office for Europe in Copenhagen next week. If there is not a major improvement in my support I will resign.

My speech at the 42nd Meeting of the Regional Committee of WHO for Europe 15th September proved to be a turning point. It was an unscheduled intervention in the sense that it did not appear on the programme and was kindly permitted at my request by the Chairman. It was a success, perhaps the most successful speech I have ever made. It was obvious that it came from the heart. Indeed the Slovenian minister who I had recently met in Ljubljana and was present said it 'exposed my soul.' That I was congratulated not only by the Croat and Bosnian Ministers but also by the Serb Minister must be almost unique. The Croat Minister complained that I was wrong to speak of parts of Serbia as being damaged by the war. But in spite of the fact that he said rightly that "there are no windows broken in Serbia", there are tens of thousands of penniless refugees there who need help and also many injured people.

During the remaining days of September, money and promises of money flooded in. By the end of the month I had funds not only for major programmes of humanitarian relief but for properly furnished and staffed offices in Zagreb, Sarajevo, Belgrade, Split and Skopje in Macedonia. Most of important of all, as the last of the autumn leaves were falling and the air was chilly, WHO's Copenhagen office was able to send me the Finnish Army's senior expert in Low Temperature Survival, Lt. Col. Risto Tervahauta.

Risto Tervahauta

"It was the last Friday of November 1992 when my superior from Helsinki telephoned me. WHO has inquired whether Finland could find a medical officer with experience of working in war zones and knowledge in low temperature medicine. He would be invited to run a winter survival project for Sarajevo which was heading towards

winter under siege and with a serious lack of heating, gas, electricity and water. Some 300,000 people were in danger of freezing and the city was under continuous shelling.

The task did not sound very attractive! However, I telephoned the WHO Copenhagen office and heard that if I hesitated a Swedish Major was ready to go. In view of the historic differences between Finland and Sweden, this settled the matter for me and any doubts I may have had vanished. I had no choice but to accept the mission and I flew to Copenhagen on the Monday and was in Zagreb on Tuesday evening."

On the 4th December 1992, the date on which I welcomed Risto into my office in Zagreb was a 'Red Letter Day' in WHO's mission to the Former Republic of Yugoslavia. From that date, until shortly before the mission closed down, we had at our disposal not only a low temperature survival expert but a trained soldier. Within a few days, our offices and convoys were organised so that we stopped taking unnecessary risks and worked more effectively. He prepared two important papers for us. How to stay alive and how to keep warm. Firstly, when under fire make yourself as small as possible and keep still. Secondly, put on as much clothing as you can find and keep dry. Sounds obvious doesn't it – but I nearly lost one of my colleagues who did not.

I also remember two points in particular from our first conversation. The first was that he had already skied one hundred kilometres across country in Finland that autumn. The second was the gentle way he broke some bad news. This was that the consignment of black plastic bags which someone in London in the Polar Expedition Group had foisted on me for use as sleeping bags for refugees in the open, while okay at the North Pole, these were useless (due to condensation) in a damp climate. This is because the first rule of survival in sub-zero temperatures is to keep dry! They therefore quickly reverted to their original role as bin-liners.

But if, as the years pass the memory of Risto's work in FRY (Former Republic of Yugoslavia) fades among his former WHO colleagues, there is a small town in a remote part of Bosnia where he will not be so easily forgotten. Zepa is one of the Moslem towns – like Srebrenica – which suffered because it was close to the Serbian border. In this case the Serbs blocked the road at both ends of the village and left the people to starve. Risto reconnoitred the area on skis and by his superb field craft discovered a forgotten path through the forest. This was secretly reopened and sustained the population of Zepa for the rest of the war.

2nd January 1993

The biting cold at Sarajevo airport (-12c at 7am) made our toes, ears and noses sore within a few minutes as we walked from the Hercules aircraft to our car. The crucial issues here are not only the effect of the lack of fuel of all kinds upon the capacity of people to keep warm, but also the lack of electricity for pumps which has effectively destroyed the public water supply. The available water now comes from the well at the brewery distributed by fifteen U.N. water tankers. There are long queues, and we saw many people of all ages walking to water distribution points with pails at the same time risking sniper fire.

The current situation was confirmed to me by Major Manfrais of the French army. Lack of electricity makes it impossible to pump water in central heating systems so that gas fired furnaces for blocks of flats cannot be used but those lucky enough to have a neighbour with a wood burning stove congregate in one room and live from day to day on what they can find.

A surgeon at the State Hospital described how he wakes up with his face frozen each morning in spite of covering himself as best he can with all available blankets. Another doctor, who walks up and down when he is on duty at night in his overcoat to stop himself shivering, said as the weeks passed and the shortages of food and fuel became critical they would "fight each other like animals if necessary to survive but would never leave." Without heating he would not be able to treat frostbite or hypothermia.

We went to a Refugee Centre which shelters several hundred women, children and men unfit or too old for military service. The corridors and toilets were filthy and it was bitterly cold. In one room with a makeshift wood burning stove there were five people including an ex soldier whose wound gave him privilege of a supply of fuel. In another room there were three elderly people, one almost blind who had been displaced from Foca, but the room in this case was reasonably warm simply because it faced south, there was double glazing and there had been sunshine all day. Although they had lost everything they considered themselves lucky to be alive!

Some people we stopped to talk to in the street expressed their anger about the hypocrisy of the UN in permitting the situation to arise. They felt deserted.

3rd *January*

Having consulted Risto, I have decided to insist that as long as the severe weather continues that high quality blankets and sleeping bags must take priority over food on the airlift. But my colleagues in

UNHCR conclude that I have taken leave of my senses. In plain terms the logic is that while sub zero temperatures in the absence of heated buildings or adequate clothes/blankets will kill in hours, death from starvation takes weeks. After hours spent in argument to no avail I have finally got my way!

4ᵗʰ January

A wonderful day.

(1) *20,000 high quality sleeping bags have arrived in Zagreb and they are being packed for urgent despatch to Sarajevo by airlift. More are on the way.*

(2) *An armoured Land Rover to replace my current 'soft' vehicle has arrived from Provence – why Provence of all places?*

(3) *After six months in the field WHO has at last provided me with administrative support: an ex-warrant officer in the British Army to manage our warehouse and an experienced Swiss journalist to act as my Press Officer are on the way.*

I reflect that if in the coming months anything should happen to any of my people I can at least say that I have asked no one to do anything which I have not been prepared to do myself.

I also managed to lead a convoy to Tesanj, the remote Bosnian town from which within a few days of my arrival the two medical brothers had come to my office to seek help. It was a long and difficult journey for us through the forest and not without risk. To our dismay as darkness was falling we at last reached our destination and found ourselves far from welcome. Of the brothers there was no sign. And as for those who met us:

"You should have got to us months ago," they said.

Not surprising due to this attitude there was no room for us at the inn. We collapsed into sleeping bags on the stone floor of the clinic. Anyway, they announced it was weapons and ammunition they needed not food or medical supplies. A bitter and disheartening moment indeed. What an ironic turnaround! For more than any other factor, it had been the testimony of the medical brothers from Tesanj that they were operating without anaesthetics, in an unheated theatre and that the women and children were now dangerously thin which during the preceding months had inspired and spurred me on in my work throughout Bosnia.

The Post-Traumatic Stress Disorder
Another aspect of the humanitarian relief effort in FRY pointed to the UN's lack of experience in this type of work. No guidelines had been issued on the need for personnel to take regular leave. After I arrived I noted that some colleagues who had been daily taking risks and who had also witnessed appalling tragedies were on the edge of mental breakdown. We therefore instituted a system of compulsory leave breaks of at least two and preferably four weeks every three months for our staff. We also made available de-briefing sessions by a trained psychologist as soon as one became available.

A few days later, almost as if Risto's arrival had been magical, the weather changed and Sarajevo had an unusually mild spell. But when in February the snow returned the widely distributed sleeping bags, blankets and wood burning stoves paid off and saved many lives.

In the remaining weeks of my tour of duty I made my eighth and final visit to Sarajevo. On this occasion I managed to recross the line and visit the suburbs of Sarajevo outside the siege. Ironically, as the whole country was in chaos, the besiegers were also starving and their needs seemed as great as the besieged. For me, nothing underlined the futility of the Bosnian civil war more heavily than this.

CHAPTER 3
Ulster Childhood

I have two indelible memories of the house in Belfast in which I was born. The first is of the lamplighter who managed to light the gas lamp outside our gate with his long pole without stopping to get off his bicycle each evening. However much he wobbled he never fell off. The second is when an Indian wigwam in which I was sitting in the garden with my toys collapsed. In spite of my howls, although it was probably only seconds, it seemed an age before anyone came to my rescue. Hence, no doubt, my life long claustrophobia.

My paternal ancestors came from Scotland but early in the seventeenth century moved to Ireland in the Plantation of Ulster. They were granted land in County Armagh where they put down roots as yeoman farmers. They evidently prospered for my great grandfather became a clergyman and my grandfather, David Acheson, served in the Royal Navy as a paymaster during the American Civil War. According to family tradition, his ship cruised off New Orleans with the British fleet to protect the export of cotton from the Confederate States to the mills of Lancashire. Perhaps this convinced him of the importance of textiles, for on retiring from the Navy he returned to Ulster and used his bounty to found the family linen weaving business in Castlecaulfield, Co. Tyrone. It was into his house, still occupied today by his descendents that in 1882 my father was born.

In a family such as ours that had a tradition of late marriage, ancestral memories are long. Thus I have a clear memory from childhood of my grandmother, Sarah Acheson, although she was born in 1855 nearly one and a half centuries ago. I used to be brought to tea with her after my weekly music lesson. She wore a long black dress with a white lace cap and a black widow's band round her neck. Her fingers seemed very thin and bony and her rings rattled on the piano keys as she played *'Annie Laurie'*.

When the family went to the seaside at Castlerock on the north coast of Ireland for the summer holidays, our car a Riley 'nine', was too small to cope with all of us so, being the youngest I used to go by rail with Grannie. As she was a very punctual person, to be certain we would catch our train, she insisted that we should arrive at the station in time to see the train before our train to Castlerock draw out. So, for what seemed like an age, we sat solemnly side by side in the waiting room at the Midland station in Belfast, she in her black bonnet and coat and I with my legs dangling beside her.

My parents

My mother came from the north of England. She was born in South Shields on Tyneside. The Rennoldsons had originally been the millers of Jesmond Dean but in the nineteenth century, as industry in the Northeast developed, they prospered. From millers, in successive generations they became first millwrights, then shipwrights, and finally shipbuilders.

Even allowing for the greater uncertainties of life as it existed a century ago, my mother had a harrowing childhood about which she rarely spoke. Soon after her favourite sister Alice had died of consumption, her mother developed breast cancer for which she suffered no less than twelve operations. These, as was the custom among the well-to-do in those days, were conducted not in hospital but at home, sadly in her case to no avail. Then in my mother's late teens her father, to whom she was very close, developed diabetes. For want of insulin which had not yet been discovered, he also died. Looking back I wonder whether these tragedies left an indelible mark so that when she herself became a mother she sometimes found it difficult to express to us the love she felt.

My maternal grandfather, Joseph Rennoldson, the Tyneside shipbuilder, made such a success of building paddle-powered tugs that they were exported widely throughout the Empire. One of them, the 'Lady Brassey', was still in service in Dover in World War II and took part in the Dunkirk evacuation. Grandfather Rennoldson also took up local politics for the Liberal Party and in 1896 became Mayor of South Shields.

There is a romantic story about how my parents met. As Joseph Rennoldson was a widower living alone, it was decided to send young Dorothy to a finishing school in Hampstead to learn the social graces. There she met a number of young ladies of like background who became lifelong friends. One of these, Nan Swan, was the daughter of a Dundee jute textile manufacturer who had links with my grandfather's linen business in Castlecaulfield. The relationship blossomed and I have a photograph of the wedding in 1910 between my father's younger brother Vincent and Nan Swan at which my father was best man. My mother, as yet unmarried, was also present. Soon afterwards another friend from Birklands, Dorothy Low, married a second Acheson brother, my father's elder brother Frank. Finally, in 1920, my mother married a third brother. This was Malcolm Acheson, a doctor who was to become my father.

I was close to my father and even now, more than forty years after his death, feel his influence. At Dungannon Royal School to which he trudged daily the two and a half miles across the fields from

Castlecaufield, his talents both on and off the playing field were soon spotted. He was coached for entry to Trinity College, Dublin, into which he passed with Merit to read medicine in 1901. In the same year, among his classmates was the first woman in the British Isles to be admitted to a university to study medicine. While in due course other medical schools followed suit, prejudice against women students died hard and for many years female medical students remained a small minority. Even seventy years later when I was Dean of the new medical school at Southampton, I had to fight hard to get agreement that there should not be a 'quota' for women but that places should be awarded to men and women equally on merit without regard to gender.

But another aspect of my father's experience as a medical student was to have a greater and more pervasive influence on my life. This derived from his opinion that an exclusively science-based course at school was too narrow to be suitable preparation for a career as a doctor. In his own case he had concentrated on Classics prior to entry to Trinity and in the first year of the medical course had taken Liberal Arts (logic, ethics, philosophy, etc.) in parallel and had achieved Honours. When I made my own decision to become a doctor, to the consternation of my teachers in Edinburgh, my father's priorities for me differed sharply from theirs. He insisted that in the Sixth Form I should take History and English, not Chemistry and Physics – expressing himself confident that I could 'catch up on science' later.

And so it turned out that when I left school I had a simple model of the outline of English and European History since the Reformation. As for English literature, in addition to the Prologue of the Canterbury Tales and the Tempest, I had read some Tennyson and Browning as well as Vanity Fair and Nicholas Nickleby. How, if at all, this unusual experience affected my skills as a clinician I do not know, but I am certain it has had a major influence of my enjoyment of life.

Perhaps because being a doctor seemed such a settled part of his life, I do not remember asking my father why he opted for a medical career in the first place. One story has it that it was simply to guarantee an opportunity to play rugby at University level for five seasons. This indeed he achieved and more, for in addition to representing TCD for four years, he played for Leinster against the All Blacks on their first tour and gained a trial cap for Ireland.

If sport was indeed his initial motive for becoming a medical student, the encounter with disease and death in the medical course changed him as it has many others before and since. Overcrowding and malnutrition were rife in the Dublin of his day and as a medical student their consequences were everywhere to be seen. At the Richmond Hospital he encountered tuberculosis, which was epidemic in Ireland at that time in all its forms. Diphtheria was also rampant and he soon became adept at performing emergency tracheotomy - the lifesaving operation which involves cutting open the windpipe in the neck and inserting a breathing tube for children choking with the membrane of the disease. In my teens, I remember him showing me how this was done with my neck extended over the back of a chair and his finger drawing a vertical line on my throat.

My father's clinical training also brought him, as it did myself fifty years later, to experience domiciliary obstetrics in Dublin's slums. There was no hope that the techniques of the day could counter the consequences of poverty, uncontrolled fertility and the lack of antenatal care. Infant mortality was high. This experience together with busy junior posts in surgery, medicine and bacteriology took their toll. Within a short time of qualifying as a doctor he not only developed one of the less serious forms of tuberculosis but also became the first patient in Ireland to be operated on for a bleeding duodenal ulcer. Fortunately for him, bearing in mind that in those days blood transfusion was not available, he not only recovered but remained free of symptoms for more than thirty years.

When in 1909 my father moved to Liverpool to set up his plate as a general practitioner the epidemic of syphilis that was sweeping Europe was at its height. In a city, which at that time was one of the busiest seaports in the world, the disease in all its forms was rife and he became expert in its treatment. The emphasis he gave to the need for absolute secrecy in caring for patients with 'venereal diseases' – even in the extreme instance of a husband and wife who unwittingly had come separately to see him and would not give consent for the other to be informed – made a lasting impression on me. Many years later this insistence on strict confidentiality to encourage patients with sexually transmitted diseases to come forward for speedy diagnosis and treatment led me to insist it should become the cornerstone of the British government's policies on AIDS.

Fortunately 1911 saw the arrival on the market of a drug derived from arsenic (salvarsan), which proved lethal to the spirochete which causes syphilis, and revolutionised the treatment of this dreaded disease. Salvarsan turned out to be the first of the 'magic bullets' combating infections which were invented in the twentieth century and of which penicillin and streptomycin are more recent examples. These proved so effective that it soon became possible to close a host of hospitals and many thousands of beds devoted to the treatment of tuberculosis, syphilis and other infectious diseases.

I still have my father's notebook on treatment written in his own hand which, almost one hundred years ago, he carried with him on his rounds as a general practitioner in Liverpool. But how slender his resources were! Adrenaline injections for asthma (from which he himself suffered) and thyroid extract for failure of the thyroid gland had just come in. But apart from these and salvarsan and morphia for controlling pain there were only five medicines available which he believed had any measurable benefit. These were bromides for anxiety; digitalis for heart failure; iron for anaemia; quinine for people returning from the tropics with malaria and salicyclates for rheumatism.

Of father's bachelor life as a Liverpool GP, his family were told little except that as there was no rugby locally, he had turned to soccer and become a faithful supporter of Everton, treating himself after the matches to a dozen oysters at the Adelphi Hotel. He did his rounds not on foot but in a horse-drawn carriage wearing a black silk top hat and morning coat. The top hat must have been of high quality, as almost a century later it is still in use. On ceremonial occasions the hat may still be observed riding in royal processions on the head of Lord Brookeborough, Lord-in-Waiting to the Queen, the husband of my niece and one of my father's granddaughters.

As father was a somewhat shy and retiring person, it is possible that he may have been celibate during his time as a GP in Liverpool or there may have been relationships of which his family never heard. Fortunately it was easy for him to step on the overnight Belfast ferry at Prince Albert dock and breakfast with his mother next morning. In 1910 and 1911 as he passed in the steamer up Belfast Lough, he could not have missed the huge hull of the *'Titanic'* taking shape in the shipyard of Harland and Wolff. A few years earlier, in 1905, according to family tradition, he and his brother Frank had taken delivery in Belfast docks of one of the first batch of cars to be imported to Ulster. Then with great difficulty they drove it over bumpy unmetalled roads to Castlecaulfield for my grandfather's use.

But events were shortly to take place which not only led my father to bid farewell to Liverpool, but shattered the lives of tens of millions of people and changed the course of history. On 28 June 1914 in Sarajevo, Archduke Franz Ferdinand of Austria and his wife were assassinated by a Serb nationalist. Within six weeks Germany had invaded France and a British Expeditionary Force was on its way to Flanders. Father's response was immediate. He boarded the London train at Lime Street, took a taxi to Millbank and applied to join the Army as a medical officer. But in spite of the fact that, in his own words, he was able not only 'to operate, give an anaesthetic and use a microscope but also ride a horse', to his bitter disappointment he was turned down. This was because (of all things) his teeth were regarded as inadequate. Two weeks later when the German army was almost at the gates of Paris he tried again. By this time, not surprisingly, although his dental condition had not changed, attitudes had and he was welcomed with open arms. By mid October 1914 he was in France, spending his first night in comfort in the Grand Hotel Moderne in Le Havre. This according to its surviving letterhead proudly provided *'chauffage central, ascenseur, electricité, et l'eau chaude et froide.'* But it was in Flanders in very different circumstances save for an intermission of six months in 1917 that he remained as a volunteer for the rest of the war.

Letters From France

During the war years, father wrote regularly from France to his mother who by this time was widowed. Some of the letters have survived and help us appreciate the appalling conditions under which doctors in the Royal Army Medical Corps had to work in that war. In the absence of antibiotics, blood transfusions or other intravenous fluids, a high proportion of the wounded died. In the early days when my father was serving at a base hospital he had to cope not only with wounded but outbreaks of both typhoid fever and diphtheria. Tetanus and gas gangrene were also rife and he described whole wards set aside for the care of these two deadly conditions. At the door of the tetanus ward was the sign 'SILENCE'. The slightest sound would precipitate a veritable epidemic of agonising tetanic spasms among the patients. As for the gas gangrene ward, it could be smelt a hundred yards away. In those days the only treatment available for shock was hot, sweet tea and even that could not be given if the wound had penetrated the abdomen. Fortunately, thanks to the introduction of anti tetanus serum and more careful splinting of damaged limbs, there was a steady reduction in overall fatality rates. For stretcher cases these fell from 28% in 1914 to 8% in 1918.

After six months service in the comparative safety of a Base Hospital where he doubled up as a bacteriologist and anaesthetist, father arranged to be posted to a Field Ambulance which was supporting the First (Guards) Division. As this was close to the Front Line, conditions were far from comfortable. A letter to his mother written in July 1915 shortly after his arrival speaks for itself:

First Field Ambulance
First Division
30/7/15

> *My dear Mother,*
>
> *Yes, I liked the assortment of good things [you sent] very much...*
> *Have a fair amount of work with every other night on duty. Insects*
> *here are a most dreadful pest, flies, mosquitoes and vermin generally.*
>
> *...We have all the sick and wounded of a division which is in action to*
> *look after. It is deplorable to see some of these fine chaps who are*
> *brought in mortally wounded.*
>
> *One of our sergeants went out to bring in some of 'the boys' who were*
> *stupid enough to be watching an aeroplane in an exposed position and*
> *got it in the neck. Nobody else did.*
>
> *Glad to read Lloyd George's speech and the promise of better things to*
> *come contained therein.*
>
> *The fly trap on the table in front of me which was empty an hour ago*
> *contains about 300 flies and I don't think I'm exaggerating. You can*
> *imagine the state of the room...*
>
> *I wonder could you get me a couple of Khaki cotton – not flannel*
> *...[shirts] with 16½ inch necks.*
>
> *The weather is too hot [here] for a town under war conditions.*
>
> *Your affectionate son,*
> *M.K.A.*
> *[Malcolm King Acheson]*

But as time went on, due no doubt to the cumulative effect of the suffering he had witnessed, my father's style changed. It became direct and explicit and spared his mother nothing. Here are two word for word extracts, the first describing how he received a leg wound on September 1st 1918, the second on his reflections on returning to duty:

> "Perhaps you would like to know how it happened. Very hot day a month ago – mouth of a dugout – about 30 helpless patients blinded by mustard gas – the process of their being stripped of their contaminated clothes and put in pyjamas – lorry waiting to take them to next Dressing Station – 200 yards away a shell large size explodes – overhead a Hun 'spotting' plane – tremendous haste of willing RAMC orderlies – 150 yards away another shell – more frantic haste – lorry filling, driver impatient – 100 yards away another shell – tearing, sweating haste to put patients in lorry now ¾ full – 50 yards away a shell, splinters, bricks, dust. – Lorry driver soundly cursed twice for starting without my orders – lorry goes 'at the double' – orderlies and 3 patients returning to dugout. Crash, stars, blow in leg – voice "He's done for."
>
> But he wasn't! I can now get about on a stick and am little the worse."[11]

The second letter was written a few weeks later just before the Armistice ended the war on 11th November. In it he describes a deserted battlefield he visited on a walk near his place of convalescence from which the fighting had moved on:

> "This is a barren waste. I hadn't realised until today what it was really like. Huts riddled and scorched with dismal flapping roofs. Miles of rusty barbed wire overgrown with rank grass; old shell

---

[11] Letter from MKA to his mother from 1. Field Ambulance 2/11/18.

holes half filled with yellow ooze; stark telegraph poles with wires streaming and sighing in the wind; overgrown trenches filled with helmets, mud boards, bones; graves galore; bricks where villages stood; wrecked bridges built and built again; heaps of tins, old cartridges; rusting shells, boots, clothes torn to shreds and filth. The tracks of camps old and new: dugouts and shelters – in a word, a country devastated and seared with war."

He sums up with a final comment:

"This must have been a lovely part of France beside the fatal river – the Somme, the name of which will in future always bring to mind a vision of what Hell may be like."

In 1916 two years earlier on that very same river, my father had been awarded the Military Cross for his work in bringing in the wounded at Highwood in the 'Valley of Death.' According to the citation the decoration was for

"Conspicuous gallantry and devotion to duty. He tended the wounded under very heavy fire, displaying great courage and determination. By his devotion and initiative he was instrumental in saving many lives."[12]

Just one week later by a tragic turn of events his younger brother Vincent, an infantry officer in the Inniskilling Fusiliers serving in the Balkans, was killed trying to ferry wounded soldiers in his Company

---

[12] Supplement to the London Gazette 14 November 1916 p11045

across the swollen river Struma. I have often wondered whether the same post brought the news of these two events to my grandmother.

Against all this sound and fury of which in so far as I understood my father's role, I felt pride at a respectful distance, but there was another father I loved with all my heart. I present a vivid cameo of him in later life. We are now living in London where the family had moved in 1936 as his career in the Civil Service advanced. His senior colleague at the Ministry of Pensions throws a party for him and we are all invited to a formal dinner. I am ten and this is the first time I have had an evening meal away from home. In addition to my parents and myself our host has brought his own family. As we sit down I find that for some reason each of us has three glasses and a puzzling array of knives and forks. Beside me sits a girl about my own age who is the most beautiful person I have ever seen. She is our host's daughter and her name is Rose. Opposite sits my father in a white bow tie and a peculiar long black coat with tails which he has to pull up before he sits down.

Soup arrives in a huge tureen. Rose is served first and the waiter pours her soup into a strange little pot sitting in the middle of her soup plate. Not sure what to do, she begins to spoon it straight from the bowl into her mouth. But to her horror those on her right all grasp the handles carefully and upend the contents into their soup plates. Rose blushes and is just about to burst into tears. But, sitting directly opposite, my father sees what has happened, clears his throat, gives her a friendly wink and follows her example, as do the remainder of the guests.

After the war, my father entered the Ministry of Pensions in Belfast as a medical officer. As his task was to supervise the care and support of

Ulster ex-servicemen disabled in the World War, he was in a sense thereby continuing the work he had begun in France.

Many years later when I was leading the WHO Relief Programme in Bosnia, something occurred which reminded me of the events which had happened at Highwood and in the Dardanelles on the Struma River in 1916. One of my team, a young surgeon called Simon Mardel, having managed to get to Srebrenica when it was besieged and under attack by the Serbs, set up a makeshift operating theatre illuminated by power generated by rotating a bicycle wheel. The inhabitants, by this time mostly women and children, noticed the arrival of some United Nations peacekeepers in armoured cars. Thinking they would be saved they rushed to the vehicles. At this point the Serbs opened fire and many of the civilians fell dead or wounded. Exposing himself to considerable danger, Simon went to their aid and did what he could for them for several hours without regard to his own safety. The citation describing his actions for which he was awarded the OBE bears a remarkable resemblance to my father's citation for his MC.

Katie McCallum

The other person in my childhood who has had a profound and lifelong influence on me was my nurse, Katie McCallum. Katie, who came from Portaferry in Co. Down, and arrived to look after me when I was thirteen months old. She stayed for more than fifty years. Until I went to boarding school she was an inseparable companion, supervising my meals and daily walks and nursing me through my illnesses. The fact that she was with us at all was a tribute to my parents' tolerance, for in Belfast in those days - because a social lesion festered there - it was almost unheard of for a Protestant family to employ a Roman Catholic.

Whatever the neighbours in that bitter city may have thought, probably because of my father's reputation, no one dared say a word.

As it was, Katie linked me to the other, older culture in Ulster, in which in those days there was less hope of employment and less money to go round as well as, in many cases, more mouths to feed. I now realise that in Katie's family during childhood there had been three ever present fears – hunger, unemployment and the workhouse. For many like her the only hope at that time was emigration to a new life in North America or Australia, and several of her brothers had taken that course. Although I was not aware of it at the time and she never complained, behind these social problems lay the even graver issue of religious discrimination. In the Belfast Newsletter's daily 'vacancies for employment' columns of those days, the words 'only Protestants need apply' were commonplace. No such prejudices existed in our house and one Christmas, Katie, with my parents' permission, took me to see the crib in her 'Chapel'.[13] The contrast to the seemingly drab and dull church that my parents attended still shines vividly in my mind's eye: the brightly burning candles at the altar and in the side chapels; the statues; the coloured glass in the windows and the smell of incense conveyed a glimpse of how I imagined heaven or at least fairyland might be.

Katie had grown up in a family where her mother was a widow and by the time she was sixteen she had seen two brothers die of tuberculosis. The family doctor's advice was that the best chance for Katie's health was that she should leave home and seek employment in

---

[13] So called because legislation in the 19th century had deprived Roman Catholics in Ireland of building churches with spires or towers.

England. At this interval how what followed was achieved remains a mystery. But in 1916 this girl from an obscure village across the Irish Sea was appointed as a children's nurse in the London home of the wealthy Montefiore family. Apart from having to share the family's experience of the German Zeppelin raids she was happy there. She told me how a bond of mutual respect grew up between the members of this family who for their part observed the Jewish dietary law, and Katie herself who ate no meat on Fridays and never missed Mass on Sundays.

One further small incident that occurred much later typifies this gentle soul. The fact that it remains word for word vividly in my memory shows how it affected me. In 1935 my father, now in mid-career as a medical civil servant, was posted to London and the family moved with him. My parents, Katie and I made the boat journey from Belfast to Liverpool complete with car and broke the journey at Worcester. There was time to spare and Katie and I looked into the cathedral. As we walked about we came across a royal tomb dating from the 13th century. By this time, at the age of nine, I felt I was an expert in English history.

> *"That's King John's grave, he was a wicked man and the worst king England ever had."*

Katie crossed herself.

> *"May God forgive you, Donald, for saying such a dreadful thing. There must have been some good about him, however bad he seemed. There is good in every last one of us if only our own badness will let us see it!"*

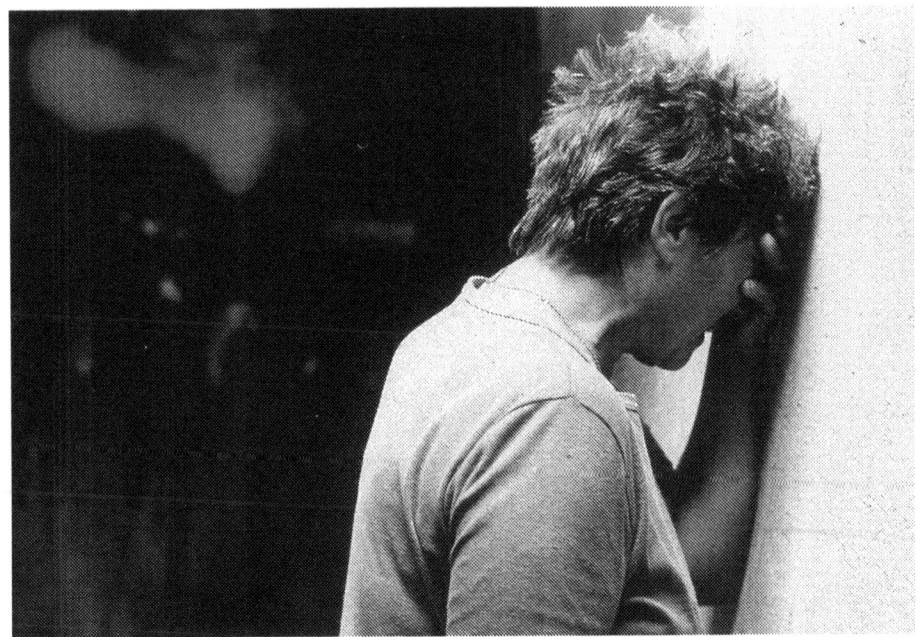

3. *Siege of Sarajevo – despair*

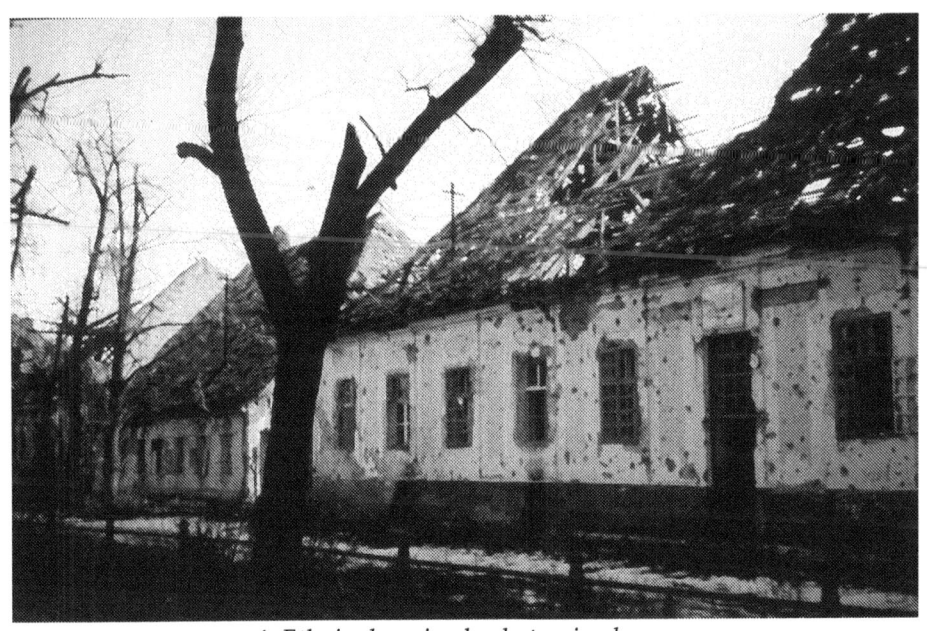

4. *Ethnic cleansing by destroying homes*

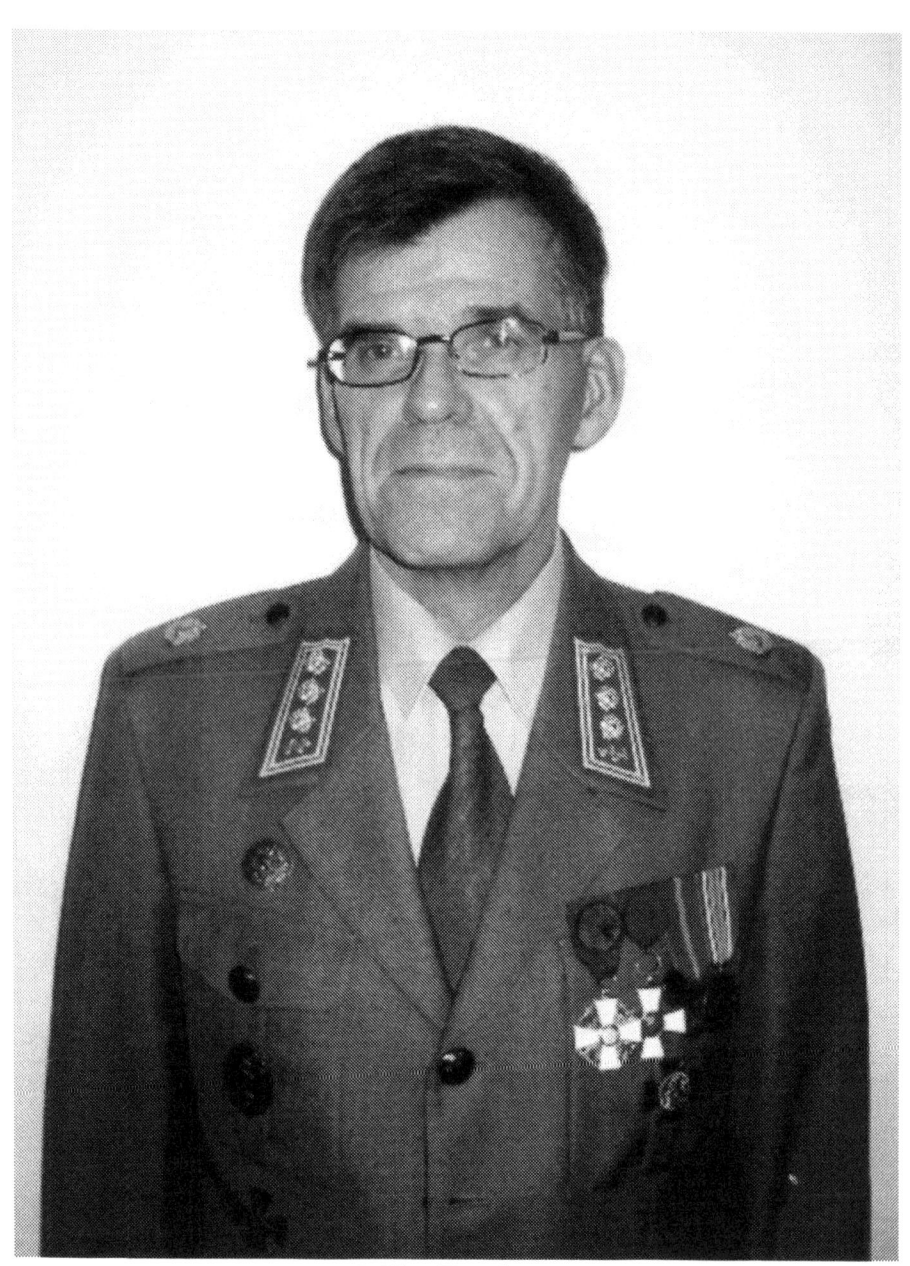

5. Risto Tervahauta

FACTORS UNDERLYING COHESION INTO GROUPS
RACE, RELIGION, CULTURE, TRIBE, COLOUR,
SOCIAL POSITION AND CIVIL UNREST

SHARED HISTORY OF PAST CONFLICT
Group A (favoured) Group B (unfavoured)

Stage 1
Unexpressed feelings
of superiority: inferiority:
social/political injustice
prejudice: fear: envy: siege
mentality: frustration

Origins
History. Education
Schools. Church
Parental Attitudes

Stage 2
Expressed as unofficial
discrimination: segregation
intimidation in jobs
housing: land ownership
All accepted by Group A
resented by Group B

Magnifying Factors
Leaders

Media
(Lennie (Riefenstahl)
"untermenschen"

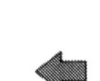

Stage 3
Sporadic unplanned outbreaks of civil unrest: riots: looting
arson: 'unofficial ethnic cleansing"

Stage 4
Premeditated policies at
national or local level involving intimidation. discrimination.
forced segregaation. and migration. ethnic cleansing

Genocide
Elimination of Group B
by Group A

2. Factors underlying cohesion into groups race, religion, culture, tribe

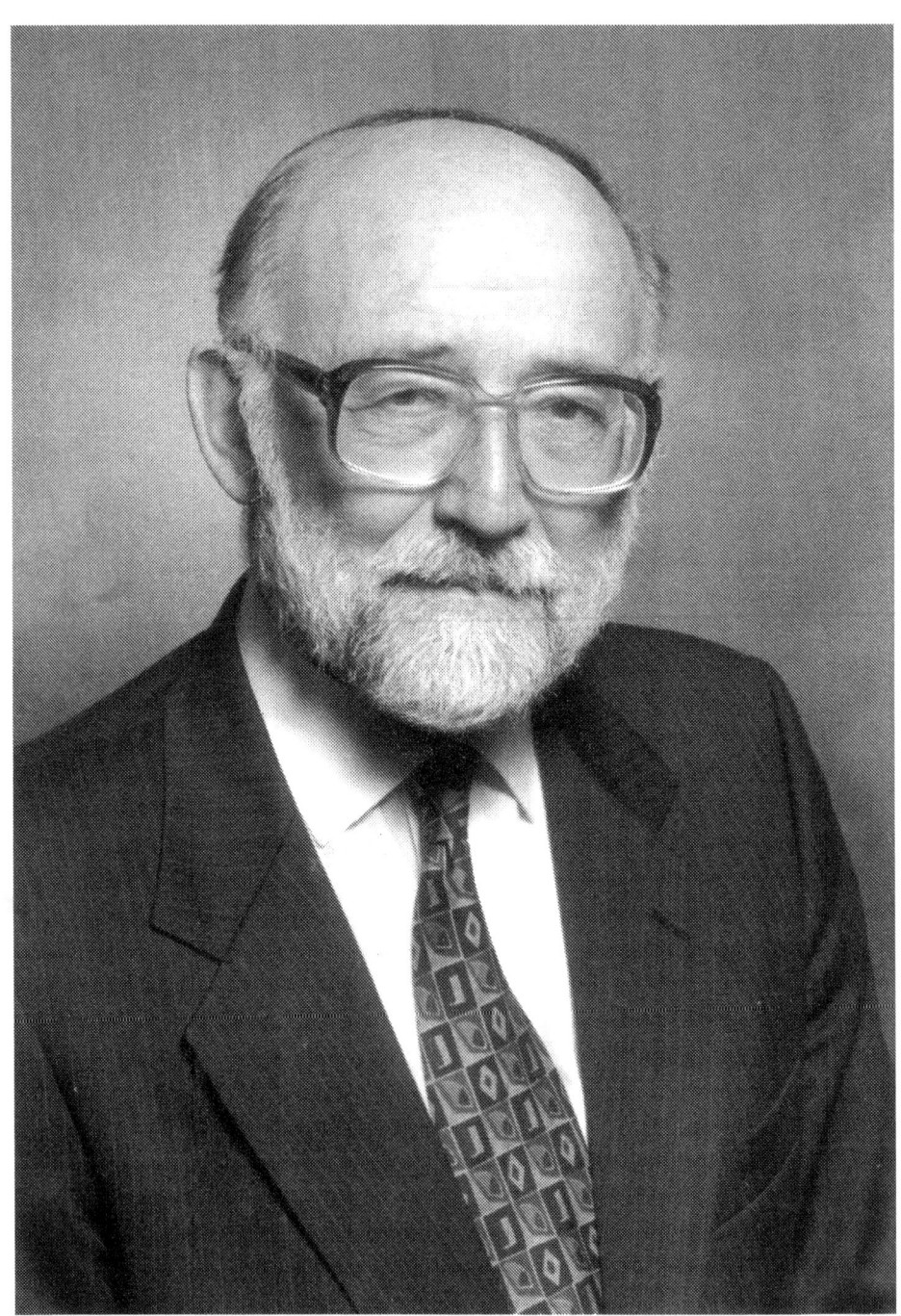

1. Sir Donald Acheson

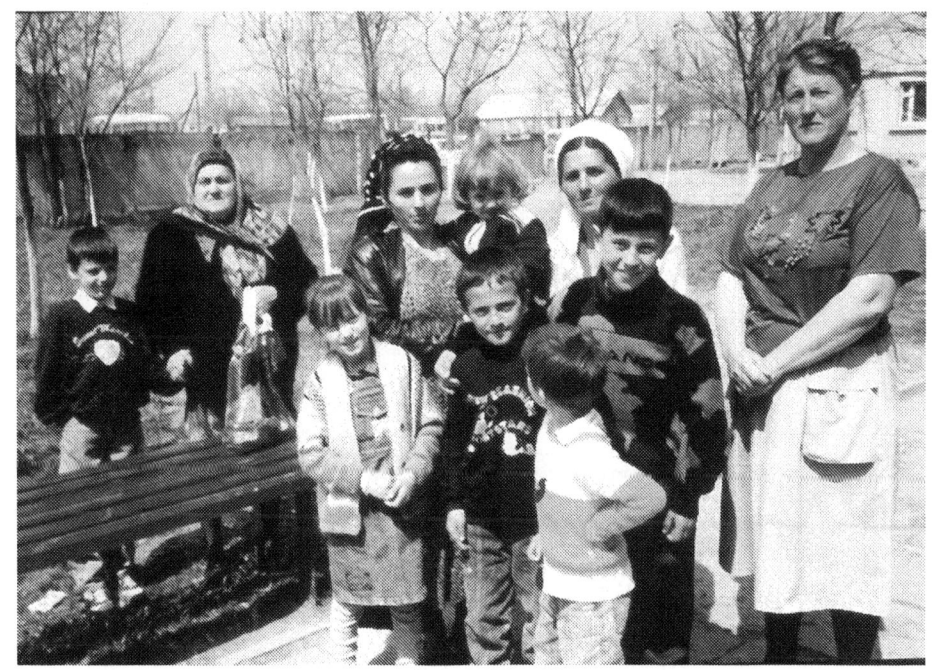

6. Displaced families

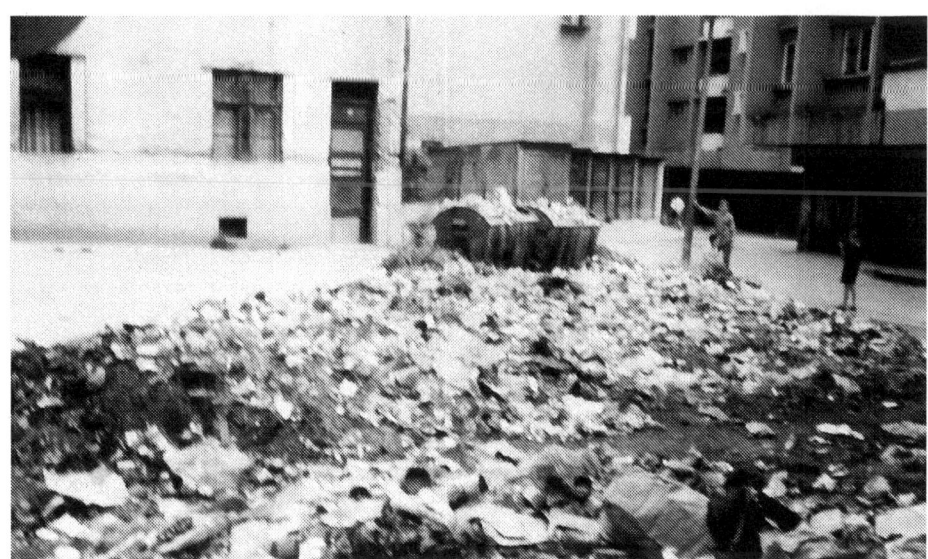

7. Sarajevo – uncollected rubbish

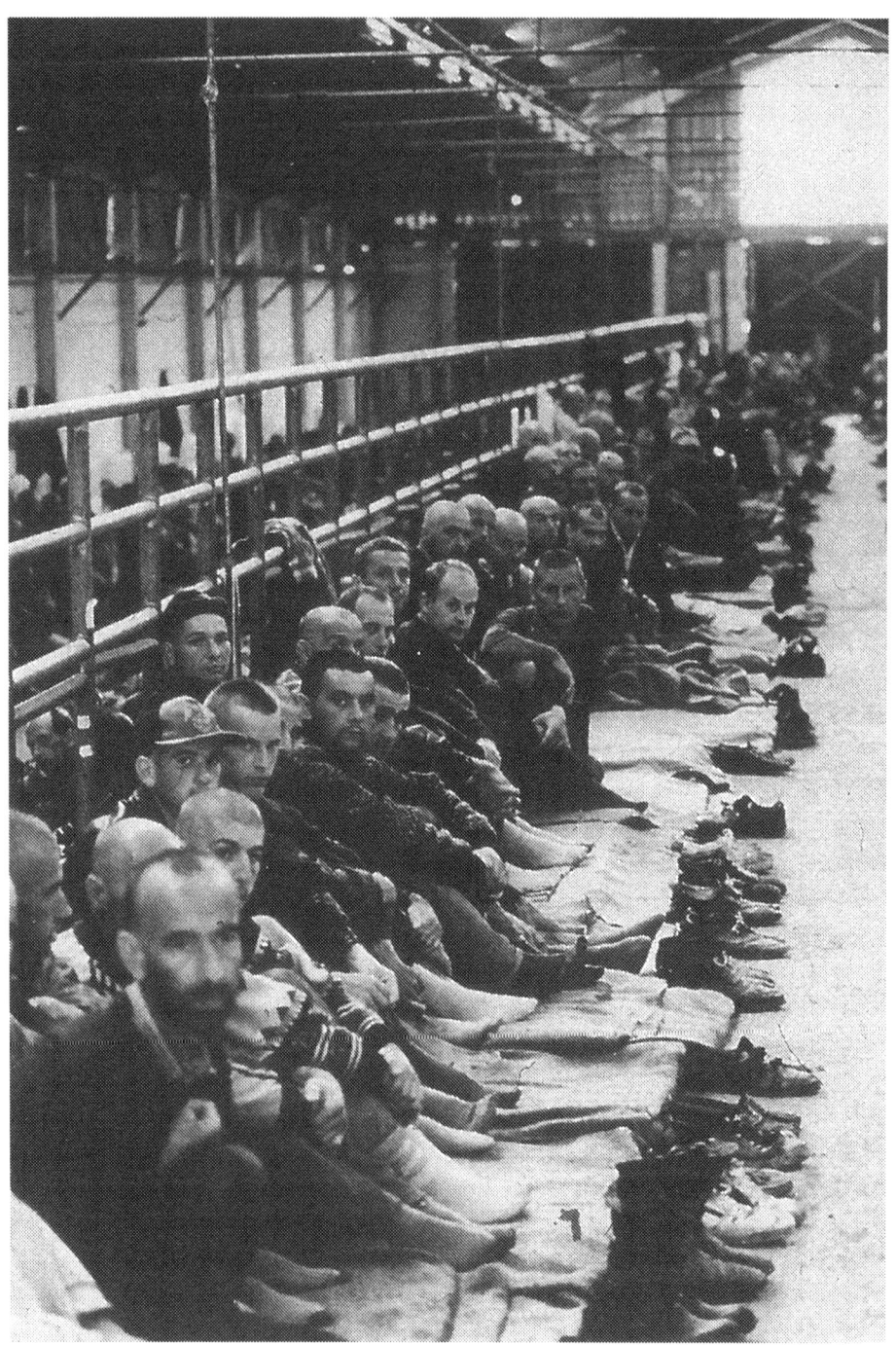

8. Prisoners of war being kept in deplorable conditions in flagrant violation of the Geneva Convention

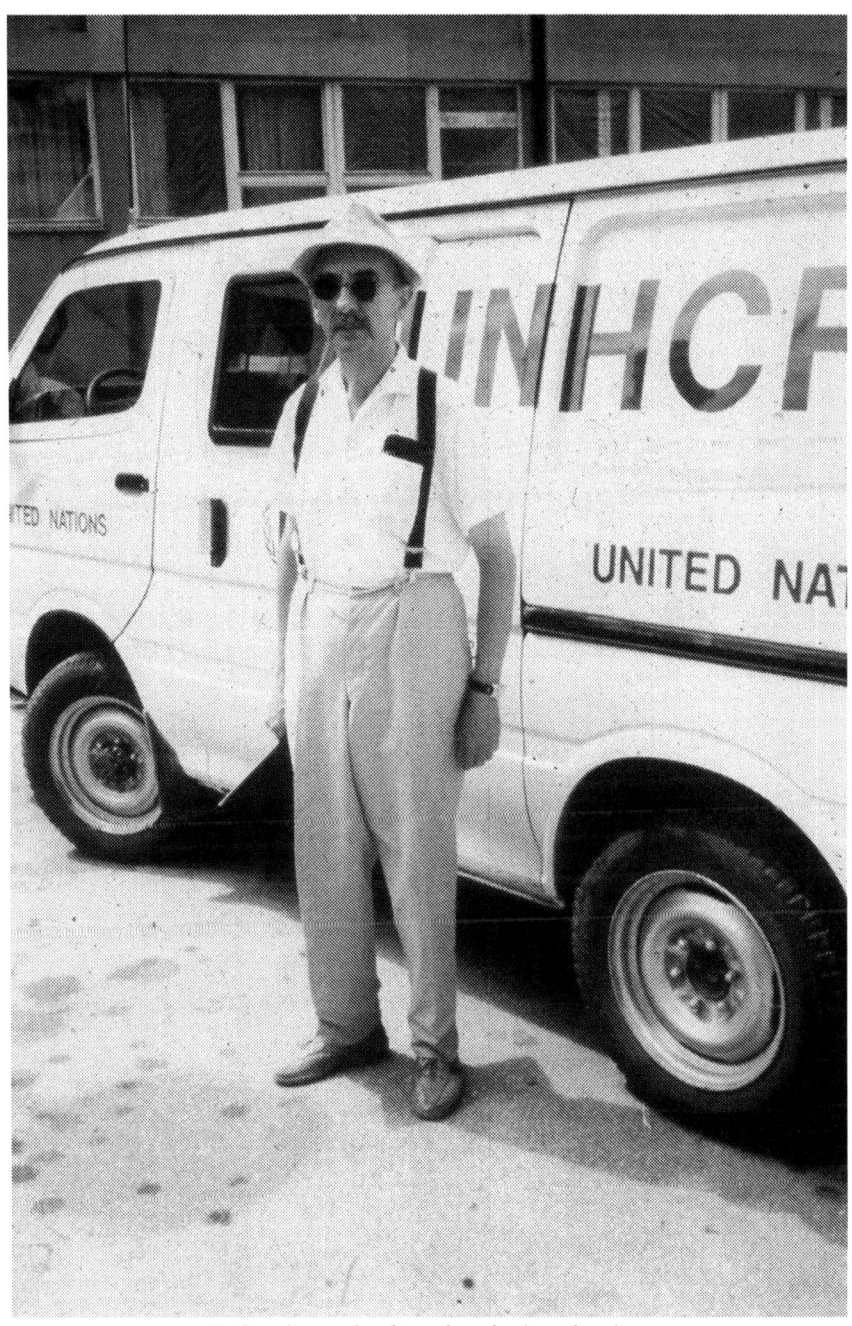

9. Sarajevo school teacher during the siege

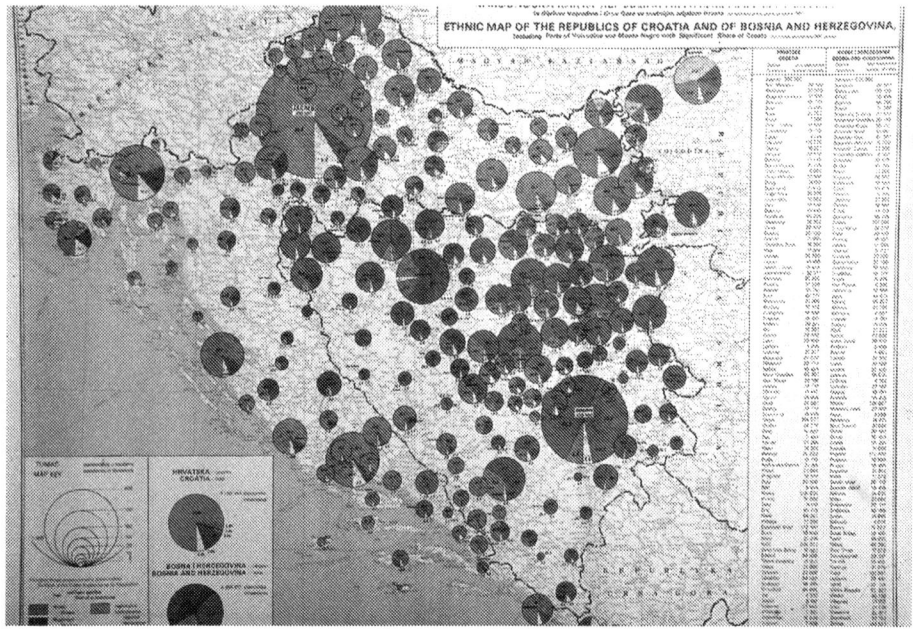

10. Ethnic map of the Republics of Croatia and of Bosnia and Herzegovina

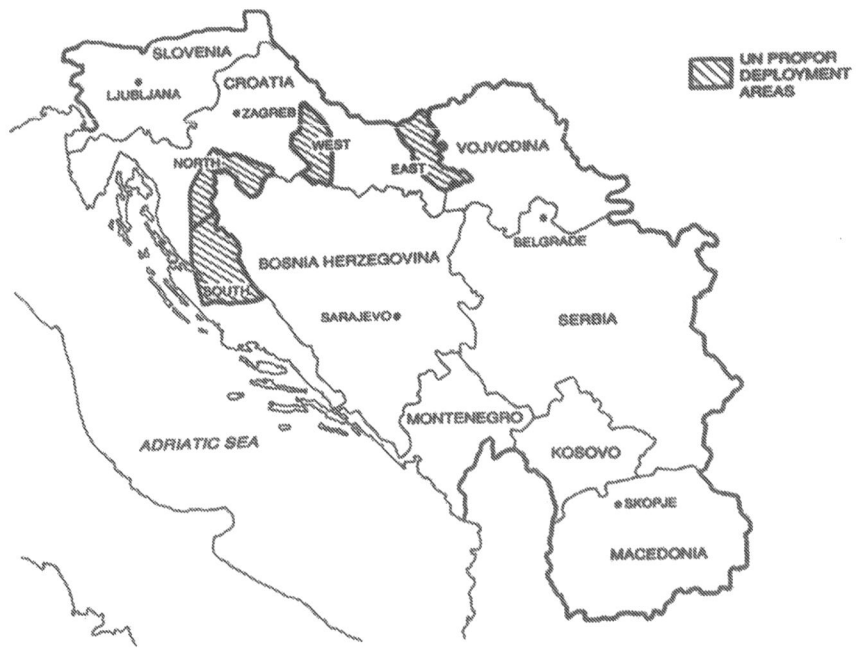

11. UN protected areas crosshatched map

CHAPTER 4
School and University

M y parents made good choices for my schooling. Not only did I learn what I needed to get me eventually to Oxford, and a career in medicine, but I enjoyed myself into the bargain. In September 1936, when I was ten and my family was living in London I was sent to a prep school at Stevenage in Hertfordshire called *'The Grange'*. The principal event which sticks in my mind is that during the Munich crisis in 1938, instead of playing cricket we were all set to work by the Headmaster, Major (the *'Beak'*) Thompson, to dig trenches to protect us against air raids. As he had been an infantry officer in World War I, these were completed in the approved zigzag pattern of that period. Happily in my time at least they were never needed.

But memory has its own system of priority. Thus it may select a happening to keep on file because it is comical or embarrassing rather than important. Such was the occasion when one fine summer afternoon the school was assembled on the cricket field for a performance of Romeo and Juliet by a group of travelling players. The staff, including the Headmaster, sat in the front row with myself, presumably because my name began with 'A', immediately behind him.

In the famous scene when Romeo and Juliet declare their love, to the horror of the Headmaster, an unscripted member of the cast began to make his appearance. What began as a gentle swelling in Romeo's tight breeches rapidly took on the unmistakable shape of an erecting penis. Unfortunately its progress was constrained so that its projection became horizontal rather than vertical. Amid muffled giggles the Beak jumped to his feet.

"You, sir, are improperly dressed!" he shouted, *"Stop the play!"*

The cast filed off amid pandemonium. Wonderfully, it seems to me now, within a few minutes all of them, Romeo included, re-emerged showing not the slightest trace of embarrassment. The play ended with a standing ovation.

The Grange had a moment of notoriety, if not fame, later when due to the war it had been evacuated to the Midlands and shared accommodation with another school. A bout of fisticuffs took place between the 'Beak' and the other headmaster, to the extent it was necessary for one of the pupils to step in and separate them. The case came to court and the pupil in question was required to give evidence. His name was Michael Heseltine, the future Conservative MP and Cabinet Minister.

At School in Edinburgh

The next step in my education was to follow my cousin and elder brother to Merchiston Castle School in Edinburgh. I arrived there from Belfast for my first term in September 1939 within a few days of the outbreak of war where by this time the family had returned from London.

During the next five years I was to sail back and forward across the Irish Sea a total of thirty times without incident. Looking back I wonder at my parents' confidence in judging that the ferries would be safe from submarine attack. Perhaps my father as a senior civil servant knew something others didn't. At any rate for whatever reason perhaps because Ireland was neutral and Germany wanted it to remain so, none of the boats although often they had British and American servicemen aboard, was attacked and I can honestly say I never felt in the slightest danger.

As we sailed down the Clyde on our way home at the end of each term, awnings were rigged in the vain hope that warships under construction would be invisible to passengers walking on the decks. After all, when the ship docked in Belfast next day, the German Embassy in Dublin would be but a three-hour train trip away. But in fact the precautions were insufficient to frustrate even a schoolboy let alone a spy. Through chinks in the awnings I remember catching glimpses of sleek blue-grey ships illuminated under a blaze of arc lights, some with guns already shipped. I now know that one of these vessels was the '*Prince of Wales*', latest battleship of the King George Vth class on which great hopes were pinned and which came to such a tragic end.

Perhaps as much because we wore shorts and open neck shirts all the year round as for any other reason, Merchiston had the reputation of being a Spartan and even a tough school but I enjoyed it. As far as homesickness was concerned, there might be salty gulp as the Irish coast and flash of the Copeland lighthouse disappeared over the horizon but next morning, as the steamer docked in the bustle of Glasgow, all such thoughts had gone.

As I look back, one benefit of my time at Merchiston has been that I have enjoyed a lifelong link with Scottish culture. Almost all the other boys were Scots – largely from professional, business or farming stock – and I soon got a taste for such delicacies as porridge, black and white pudding not to mention haggis. Although we were unaware of it at the time, at Merchiston in the 1940s as in other British public schools, we were being educated to become members of what Jeremy Paxton has called the 'Breed' – to serve the Empire. Thus many boys expected to rejoin their families in India or Africa after the war and others went into the Colonial Service. I remember an officer in the Indian Army visiting the school on what, in 1944, must have been one of the last public school recruiting drives for future officers. You could have heard a pin drop as he showed a series of lantern slides of the 'warlike tribes' – Mahratta, Sikh, Gurkha, etc. – and recounted details of recent campaigns in North Africa and on the North West frontier.

As in other boarding schools exclusively for boys at that time there was in my day at Merchiston both corporal punishment and, at least in its milder forms, homosexuality. Corporal punishment was administered on the hand by the tawse, the Scottish national instrument of correction, the number of strokes being graded by age from 'five and five' to 'ten and ten'. Usually for trivial offences such as having hands in pockets, walking on the grass, having dirty shoes or being cheeky, I both received and later as a prefect administered the tawse. Whatever the psychological consequences of corporal punishment may be, they were not recognised as adverse in those days and the system was accepted without demur by everyone – boys, staff and parents.

As might be expected when upwards of two hundred and fifty pubertal and post-pubertal lads live together without access to members of the opposite sex, emotional attachments did sometimes occur between older and younger boys. But there was at Merchiston, possibly by chance, a practical constraint that made it difficult for intimate physical relationships to develop. This was the existence within the residential accommodation of segregation by age. Thus of the four houses, Chalmers West took the entrants; Chalmers East those in the second year; while in a different building at some considerable distance

Rogerson East and West housed the senior boys. This meant that there was much less chance of intimidation or even contact between age groups than seems from the accounts of my contemporaries to have existed elsewhere.

Of sex education, if there was any at Merchiston, I remember nothing – not even of the indirect kind which in some schools is slipped in during biology classes – how the plants, the bees, the birds and the mice do it, and so on. What did happen, however, in my time was that someone imported a copy of a book called *'The Technique of Sex.'* This having circulated rapidly at a transfer fee of half a crown and become dog-eared and missing the best pages ended up inevitably in the staff common room. Even at this interval, bearing in mind that at least a quarter of us were over sixteen, what happened next seems amazing.

The following day when the whole school was assembled for roll call, the usually amiable Headmaster, Cecil Evans, known on account of his shape familiarly as 'The Tank', raised the offending book in his right hand as if he were taking an oath. You could have heard a pin drop.

"Is anyone here planning to get married in the near future?"
Silence.
"Well then! There is no place for literature of this kind in the School. Next time there will be serious trouble."

While such trivial events as these were taking place and the matter concerning us most was whether or not the School would beat its deadly rival Fettes next Saturday, we were occasionally reminded that the country was involved in a World War. Although Edinburgh itself was not a target, Rosyth, the nearby Naval Base and the Forth Bridge were, so that from time to time the sirens would sound and with the rumble of anti-aircraft guns in the distance we would all troop down to the basements for some hours of unmitigated boredom. The nearest we came to action was when within a few days of war being declared, a German bomber which had lost its way was chased over the school by a Spitfire and crashed nearby in the Pentland Hills – the first German aircraft to be shot down in the UK in the war. Some of us hoped that the next time there was a school walk in that direction, there might be something to salvage as a memento, even if it was too much to expect bodies or machine guns. But by that time, save the bent and blackened airframe, everything had gone.

It was sometime towards the end of September 1943 that I set off by train from Edinburgh to be interviewed for a place at Oxford to read medicine, hoping to begin the course in the following autumn. The trip was memorable for two reasons. The first was that London, where I had to change trains and spend the night and which for some time had been under attack by 'doodle-bugs', had just received the first of the more sinister supersonic V2 rockets, which gave no warning of their arrival. The second, which puts 'The Tank's' homily about the unsuitability for us lads of *'The Technique of Sex'* into its proper perspective, was that it was the first and last time a woman tried to seduce me in a public place.

As we rumbled out of Waverley station in Edinburgh, the train was packed with Allied service men and women. Eventually I managed to squeeze into the corner of a compartment next to a young woman wearing the uniform of the WRNS (Women's Royal Naval Service). For whatever reason – perhaps because of my extreme youth – she ignored the soldier sitting on her other side and turned her attention on me. As the train meandered slowly south through delays and diversions, her

conversation, which had begun politely enough, became first personal and finally lewd. It ended with a whispered menu of the delights I would experience if we decamped together to the WC.

In those days of sexual repression, 'sweet seventeen' was almost within the age of innocence for middle-class lads, and all this proved for me much more of an embarrassment than a temptation. I therefore did not have much difficulty in a firm 'No, thank you', whereupon she turned her attention to the soldier. As the train came to a standstill at King's Cross, the couple still had not emerged from the lavatory.

My overnight stay in London was uneventful but due to the rockets it was standing room only on the train from Paddington to Oxford. I remember nothing of the interview except that I was offered a place at Brasenose College for the following autumn, subject to my 'A' level results.

The Gleaming Spires

Although in October 1944 the tide of war had already turned, the University was still deeply affected by the conflict. The buildings themselves had escaped bombing but many of the colleges had been taken over by the armed services 'for the duration'. The students were limited to those in 'reserved occupations' such as myself or who were unfit for military service. But quite by chance the war afforded me a special privilege, which very few Oxford students over the centuries can have experienced. This was the opportunity to live for a time in two different colleges. So it was that when I arrived complete with trunk at Oxford station it was not to my own college, Brasenose, at that time occupied by the Intelligence Corps, that I directed the taxi but to Christ Church. It was there that I was to live for almost two years. Thus, although like medical students elsewhere, I worked hard in the laboratories and dissecting room, at the same time I had the joy of lodging in arguably the most beautiful College in the University, if not the world.

As might have been expected of its founder, Cardinal Wolsey, Christ Church is on a grand scale. Not only is 'Tom' the biggest quadrangle in Oxford, but the great Cardinal arranged its location so that the college or 'The House' as it calls itself, would outshine all others by incorporating nothing less than the Diocesan Cathedral itself as its chapel. Likewise the scale of the dining hall which, unchanged from Tudor times with in winter its two blazing open log fires, accommodates at least two hundred and fifty people at a sitting. But amongst this Renaissance splendour the tragic consequence of the fate which often befalls megalomaniacs is there for all to see. Instead of a closed cloister as was intended, the walkways round 'Tom' quad remain exactly as they were on the day the axe fell on Wolsey, unfinished and open to the winds.

Even towards the end of the war when I was a student of 'The House', the customs of centuries survived. Each evening, as had been the practice for more than four hundred years and indeed as it remains today, at precisely five past nine, the bell of Great Tom struck one hundred and one times; thereby to commemorate each of the students in the first class to enter the College in 1532.

But it should not be imagined that in 1944 these superb surroundings were the setting for a sybaritic existence. Far from it. In those days there was no central heating and in our rooms the coal ration barely warmed the grate. Taking a bath required a major pilgrimage across the quad come rain or shine. The food in Hall was sparse and in that time of bachelor colleges, women visitors were only permitted in the afternoons. The only consolation was that in Christ Church, at an age far too young to appreciate it, we students had access to a superb cellar. At a few pence a glass we drank wine of a quality which would have graced the table of the Athenaeum. Chateau Margaux 1934 was the first wine to pass my lips.

But the idea of going to Oxford was not for me to enjoy the scenery and taste the wine but to study medicine. The system was the same then as it is today. Most students who started at Oxford or Cambridge finished the course in London. Thus at Oxford I learned the fundamentals of biology and organic chemistry and about the structure and function of the human body and its main diseases. I then went on to the Middlesex Hospital in London to learn how to make a diagnosis and treat patients.

Institutions, however famous, have their ups and downs and Oxford and Cambridge over the centuries have been no exception. Luckily for me, immediately after the war, the Oxford medical school was at a high point and had a number of outstanding scientists. These included to mention but four: Florey and Chain, the Nobel Laureates who had identified the biochemical structure of penicillin; Le Gros Clark, the comparative anatomist; and Berenblum, whose work was unlocking the secrets of cancer. I see now that it was not the material in their lectures that mattered – within a few years even their work had passed into history. It was the self-confidence and inspiration we as students gained from being taught by people who, we realised, were working at the leading edge of science.

But there emerged from my time at Oxford an even greater benefit than that. Almost unwittingly, as it now seems, Oxford taught me how to think for myself. Even at an interval of more than fifty years, I can remember exactly when this began to occur.

It happened like this. The taxi had deposited my trunk and me at the St Aldates entrance to Christ Church and I had identified my rooms in Meadow Buildings in the farthest corner of the College. With help I had negotiated my belongings up the steep and narrow corkscrew staircase and unpacked. Suddenly I realised I had no idea what to do next. The lectures and classes probably began tomorrow – but where and when? I had seen nothing anywhere vaguely reminiscent of a classroom. The last thing I wanted to do was fail to turn up. I hurried back to the lodge. The porter seemed incongruous in his dark suit and black bowler hat but had a kindly smile.

"Yes, Mr Acheson, there is a message. Dr Percy O'Brien presents his compliments and asks if you would see him at his home on Tuesday next at 4pm."

Tuesday was five days away!

"But what am I supposed to do in the meantime?"

The porter looked at me over his spectacles:

"Settle in, sir, I should say! We've been 'ere a long time as you will have noted! I dare say Dr O'Brien will still be there on Tuesday!"

But the miracle was yet to come. When I arrived at his home at the appointed time, Percy O'Brien was solicitous and friendly. He enquired about my schooling and family background, and the comfort or otherwise of my rooms. Of biochemistry, his subject or of other aspects of the medical course he said nothing.

Then it happened, almost by the way. He looked at his watch.

"What I want you to do for me for next time is to write an essay on 'obesity'. The Radcliffe Science Library is in South Park Road. Here are some references. Not more than 2,000 words please, preferably less. The librarian will show you how the index works. The practicals and dissecting room are expensive to run so go to them but don't worry too much about the lectures. See you next week."

And then, almost as an afterthought.

"Oh! By the way, the ball's in your court now!"

And so, ever since, it has proved to be.

As the weeks went by and the friend who shared the tutorials and I read out our essays to Percy O'Brien, we were cajoled, stimulated and provoked into discussions which often extended not only well over the allocated hour but beyond the set topic. Of course, the ground we covered was not comprehensive, but if it had tried to be so it would have soon become obsolete and been overtaken by new developments. Percy O'Brien was teaching us something altogether more important: how to learn and how to think for ourselves.

Years later when in 1968 I arrived as the first Dean of the new medical school in Southampton, I did not at first find much support for this approach to teaching. Many of the staff who were already there seemed to me to have an exaggerated view of the importance of lectures, which they believed should be the backbone of the course. I called to mind the dictum of another Oxford teacher, Sir George Pickering: "a lecture is an event at which information goes from the notes of the lecturer to the notes of the student without passing through the minds of either." With the help of colleagues we pressed on.

In the end, a way was found in Southampton to develop the idea of self-learning a long step further than occurred even at Oxford. In the fourth year of the medical curriculum each student was given a period of no less than six months to formulate, develop and write up a major original project under supervision. Although in the 1970s when it was introduced, this innovation was seen as dangerously radical, after twenty-five years experience it has stood the test of time. In the earlier years of the course we also tried to ensure that the student had time for private study and self-learning. Thus the number of formal teaching hours was strictly limited to a maximum of twenty-four hours a week.

And has it so remained? Not quite! In spite of the pressure of developments in medical science undreamt of a quarter of a century ago, it has proved possible at Southampton not just to sustain this maximum of formal teaching but to reduce it further to eighteen hours. As if to prove the point about the crucial benefit of self-learning, at a recent national evaluation of all forty-two of the UK's medical schools, Southampton, after Oxford and Cambridge, came very near the top.

Brasenose College

By the autumn of 1946 the Intelligence Corps had packed its bags and BNC, with some refurbishment, was once again ready to take up its intended role. With the help of a handcart borrowed from the porter's lodge at Christ Church's Canterbury Gate I wheeled my belongings across the High Street into the College and carried them up the rickety steps of staircase VI.

While in architectural beauty BNC cannot rival Christ Church; the position of the College within the city and University is incomparable. As one looks out from the Lodge across the cobblestones of Radcliffe Square from which all traffic has recently been excluded, there is nothing visible in any direction which has not stood there unchanged for at least three hundred years. First to meet the eye is the central feature of the dome of the Radcliffe Camera with Nicholas Hawksmoor's astonishing silhouette of All Soul's College behind it; then to the right is the gothic spire of the Church of St Mary the Virgin; and to the left the 14th Century silhouette of the Bodlean Library. The benefit to the College of all this ancient masonry is practical as well as aesthetic because it creates an extraordinary silence and sense of peace within. This seems to extend beyond the ear and is a gift to scholarship.

I rarely met the student who occupied the adjacent room to mine at the top of the staircase. I knew he slept there because I heard him moving about but he had gone before breakfast and did not dine often in Hall. It was not until the middle of my second term in College that we met and chatted. It turned out that he was reading maths. His tutor who he met once a week set him a problem for each day. These he had invariably solved by 10 o'clock. He then, unknown to the College, took a train to London returning well before the College gate closed at 8pm.

The last time he and I met was at the end of our third year when both of us were receiving our B.A. degrees. He, though he had spent much of his time making a small fortune in the City, got a Double First. I fared somewhat more modestly with a 2.1. At the time I envied him not having to spend hours upon hours dissecting the human body and committing a mountain of facts to memory. But as I look back now after almost fifty years I do not think I would have willingly swapped with him even had I been able to do so.

Finally a word about the two college servants – otherwise known as 'scouts' – Bert King and Henry Bustin, who looked after me respectively at Christ Church and Brasenose. Bert, perhaps because he had a severe limp due to enemy action in World War I, had a laconic style. I can remember exactly what he said to me the first time we met.

"Good evening, Mr Acheson. I makes your bed and brings you hot water at 8 o'clock with a knock on the door. You'll find it cools quick! If you fancy a bath, it's a quarter mile walk across Tom quad."

He went on,

"And if I may be so bold as to offer advice, if you've had one, for God's sake mind the stairs. The last young gentleman nearly broke his neck; and, by the way, if you cat [vomit] on the carpet, it will cost you half a crown!"

At Brasenose, Henry Bustin, who I remember as a kind and gentle soul, also looked after the Vice Principal, Mr Platnauer, whose rooms were immediately below mine. On one occasion when I was hosting some minor celebration, a knock came at the door. There was the sturdy figure of Henry.

"Mr Platnauer sends his compliments and asks if you would kindly desist. He's fearful for his medieval ceiling."

But Henry Bustin is fixed in my memory for another reason. For it was through him that I had my first personal encounter with death. He became ill and I heard he had cancer of the gullet so I asked if I might visit him at home. Was this frail wisp who looked almost like a starved child really Henry? He could not speak. I pressed his hand. Our eyes met. I stammered something. A week later, he was dead.

CHAPTER 5

Requiem for the Middlesex Hospital

Today, anyone passing the Middlesex Hospital on the way down London's Mortimer Street might find it difficult to believe that fifty years ago it bustled with the students of one of the most famous medical schools in London. Nowadays the building is shabby and the window-frames need a coat of paint. The entrance hall is empty. The frock-coated porter who dealt with enquiries at his desk; the illuminated list of consultants currently within the hospital and the central table which displayed flowers renewed daily; all are gone. The spirit of the place echoed in the Latin motto *'miseris succerrere disco'* – I learn to care for the sick – has fled.

But when in 1948 my father, impressed by the tremendous effort which had recently gone into rebuilding the hospital by public subscription, chose the Middlesex for my clinical training, the medical school was at the peak of its reputation. I thrived there, enjoying every minute and soon found I had a flair for clinical diagnosis. I qualified in 1950 and in the succeeding years worked my way up the ladder almost to the top as a physician.

With the benefit of hindsight it now seems obvious that the Middlesex Hospital Medical School was ruined by a tragic mistake of its Board of Governors. Sometime in the middle fifties when it was already clear that there were too many medical schools and too few patients in central London, the Middlesex had the opportunity to move out to Acton. There, at Park Royal, was – and still is – an underdeveloped site and a large, overburdened hospital with a plethora of patients. Students such as myself who spent some time at Park Royal can bear witness to the matchless experience which we gained from the flow of sick people admitted to it from the surrounding multiracial community. St George's had moved to Tooting from Hyde Park Corner; the Royal Free Hospital was moving to Hampstead; why should not the Middlesex have moved to Park Royal? No doubt somewhere in the archives of its Board of Governors is buried an account of the debate which decided the issue. At the time, rumour had it that the crucial point was the convenience of the Middlesex to Harley Street. And so it may have been. After all, one can have some sympathy that senior doctors, established in their careers who, as was the custom in those days, had given their services as teachers for many years without payment, should wish to remain within a few miles of their private consulting rooms. Commuting to and from a much less convenient suburb in North London cannot have been appealing. Whatever the reason for that decision, the Medical School of the Middlesex Hospital perished more than two hundred and twenty years after its foundation in 1742. In 1968 a further reorganisation of London's medical schools took place and the Middlesex was merged with University College Hospital – as a sop, credit being given to it by retaining its name in the title of the joint school. But in the most recent reorganisation, which has united UCH with the Royal Free Hospital, except for the work of its surviving graduates, all trace of the existence of the Middlesex Medical School has finally vanished. 'Sic transit gloria mundi'!

In the 1950s when the National Health Service was barely established, there were few general practitioners in central London. The tradition was that the casualty departments of the teaching hospitals remained open day and night, seven days a week, and tried to fill the gap. Thus greatly to my benefit as a young doctor who had progressed to a senior position 'on the house' and had worked, eaten and slept there for many months, I had the responsibility of seeing patients with the spectacular range of clinical problems suffered by the polyglot local population. For our 'parish' included not only Westminster but also

Soho and contained restaurateurs, clubbers and ladies of the night as well as office workers and civil servants. One particular patient caused me so much concern and anxiety at the time that after an interval of almost fifty years I can recall every detail.

One night when I was on duty and deeply asleep, the telephone by my bed rang.

"Will you please come at once?" said an anxious voice, *"we have a serious problem!"*

I dressed and hurried to the ward. There I found a situation near to pandemonium. Everyone was awake and sitting up in bed, the lights were on and a man in his dressing gown was pacing up and down between the beds in a state of agitation. He shouted that the nurses were connected to the electric lights and trying to murder him and that he appointed all the bishops in England. Having glanced quickly at his notes and found that 'John Smith, clerk' did not correspond with the patient's grandiose account of his responsibilities, to the relief of the nurses, I sent for the 'duly authorised officer'. In those days this was the official responsible for evaluating and, if necessary, removing acutely disturbed people for treatment in mental hospitals. The DAO, as he was called, duly arrived and after all the bureaucratic processes had been completed, a sedative injection had been administered to the patient and the ambulance had departed, I went back to bed and quickly fell asleep.

But the shock that woke me the next morning was a deal greater than the one which had disturbed me in the night. Again the telephone rang but this time the voice was that of a woman.

"Are you Dr Acheson?" said an upper-class female voice, *"do you realise what you have done? My brother, who you have sent to a mental hospital, is Sir Winston Churchill's Private Secretary. How dare you do such a thing!"*

I was, I hope, polite but at that point my thoughts were a mixture of horror and disbelief. There had been, I recalled, somewhere in the great French psychiatrist Charcot's writings, reports of cases where not just one person but whole families had been affected by 'folie de grandeur'. Could this be such a case or had I made a terrible mistake?

The story ends three hours later in the civilised and relaxed office of Brigadier Hardy Roberts, the Hospital's Secretary Superintendent. Sitting with him is a second person, also smoking a cigarette in a holder and in an equally dapper dark blue pin striped suit. The Brigadier introduces him as Sir Desmond Morton from Whitehall. My heart sinks. But Sir Desmond seems kindly and asks me to sit down.

"You did exactly the right thing, Acheson," he says, *"it's really a very tragic case. What he said about himself is not far from the truth! I hope you'll get a better sleep tonight."*

At an interval of half a century when all of them are long since dead, it would be pointless to rehearse the names of the physicians and surgeons who, at the Middlesex, in the midst of their busy careers set aside valuable time to teach me the skills of clinical practice. But two, with whom I worked not only as a student but also later as a young doctor, and got to know well had a profound influence on me and must be mentioned. Douglas 'Crackers' McAlpine, was the senior neurologist, a scion of a famous family of civil engineers and, it was said, a millionaire in his own right. At a time when it was distinctly unfashionable for a London teaching hospital to interest itself in so-called 'incurable diseases', he espoused the cause of patients suffering from multiple sclerosis. At the time this was and today still remains the commonest disease of the central nervous system encountered in Britain – and one of which the mystery of its cause still remains unsolved. With invincible enthusiasm, McAlpine showed us that the degree of disability which patients suffer from MS can be mitigated not only by adapting the home and workplace to their needs but by encouragement. He was also one of the first to discover the rare benign form of MS, which does not progress. With his support I later made some discoveries about the pattern of the incidence of the disease in different parts of the world which may yet prove important. I describe these in the next chapter.

The other mentor from half a century ago whose influence I still feel was the cardiologist, Evan Bedford. Bedford, who at the time was one of the most sought after opinions on heart disease in London, was also a talented general physician. As he was never slow to remind his junior colleagues he had, when serving in the RAMC (Royal Army Medical Corp) in the Middle East during the war, successfully treated the then Prime Minister, Winston Churchill, for one of his bouts of pneumonia. But for the members of his clinical 'firm' it was his diagnosis in a very different case which brought unexpected benefits to us all. The manager of a well-known local club was admitted as an emergency to our ward at the Middlesex, having been found unconscious on the floor of his restaurant not far away. This was serious not only because it frightened the patient but also because it also frightened his clientele, who, particularly when it occurred a second time, were inclined to dine elsewhere. All the tests were negative. We were mystified. The great man stopped at the end of the bed and went over the symptoms again.

"Señor Roca, do you smoke cigars and do they sometimes make you cough?" asked Bedford.

"Si, señor" replied Roca.

"Were you coughing when you lost consciousness?"

There was a pause: yes, perhaps he had been; now he came to think of it.

"Ah!" said Dr Bedford, *"This is a case of cough syncope. Stop smoking, reduce your weight and you will have no more trouble."*

As so it was. The diagnosis of this condition, where a fit of coughing causes an overweight person to lose consciousness, was not then in many textbooks. Soon afterwards the 'Bedford firm' was entertained to a magnificent party in Señor Roca's restaurant at the Spanish Club in Cavendish Square. For months thereafter the 'House' there was open, free of charge, to the junior doctors of the firm.

I also remember Evan Bedford for the series of terse adages he offered me as advice:

"Don't earn a five- (today read 'six' for 'five') figure income before you're forty, Acheson, it's not worth the trouble in later life."

and

"Don't get on the staff as a consultant physician at too many hospitals, you'll spend your life in the car."

These were two pieces of advice about which I never had to suffer sleepless nights.

Evan Bedford's condensed clinical summaries, written in his own hand on every case he saw, covering symptoms, signs, diagnosis, treatment and prognosis and never extending beyond a paragraph, were a model I never subsequently saw equalled! But although no effort was too great to help patients with disease of the heart, Bedford's handling of those who had symptoms which they imagined were due to heart disease but had no objective evidence of it tended to be perfunctory. For these unfortunates whose illness was usually related to their personal worries, he invented a diagnosis, which I have not seen described in the textbooks – 'chronic neurotic or general ill health', abbreviated 'C N (or G) I H'. This term having been neatly inscribed in the notes together with a somewhat abrupt personal message "you have nothing the matter with your heart", the patient was returned without further ado to the care of his general practitioner with the prescription of a sedative.

But Evan Bedford's support and loyalty towards me as a young doctor, particularly on a later occasion when I was in serious difficulty, illustrates the aspect of his character I remember with particular affection. As Deputy Resident Medical Officer at the Middlesex Hospital, I shared with a colleague responsibility for decisions about admission of all patients who came as emergencies to the casualty department. One Sunday evening I was called to see a man with a number of vague symptoms who was enormously overweight and who tipped the scales at least 25 stone. After a struggle, we managed to manoeuvre him onto the examination couch. I listened to his chest but could hear nothing wrong. I then examined his abdomen and could feel nothing either. So with instructions to return the next day if he was no better, he was sent off to his home in Newman Street directly opposite the casualty department. I thought no more of him and went to bed.

Early next morning the telephone beside my bed rang. It was the police. My patient had been found dead at the entrance to his flat 'with his hat on'. In other words, he had died literally a few moments after I had examined him. What had I missed? Had I been negligent?

To cut a long story short, although I went through several days of agony, the matter ended happily – at least for me, if not for my patient. When he heard the story, my old chief Evan Bedford cancelled his appointments and, sitting side by side in the back of his huge chauffeured Cadillac, we drove together to the coroner's autopsy. In the event, I had missed nothing that could have been found by physical examination. There was no fluid in the lungs, although there was no overt coronary thrombosis, careful inspection by the pathologist showed that there was sufficient narrowing of the arteries to explain a sudden death. Was I relieved! But more than that, I was eternally grateful for the presence and personal support throughout of one of the busiest and most distinguished physicians in the land.

Obstetrics in Dublin

With its account of the slums in Limerick, Frank McCourt's recent book, '*Angela's Ashes*', reminds me of the time when in 1949, drawn by the accounts of my father's experiences half a century before, I interrupted my course at the Middlesex to learn the elements of practical obstetrics in Dublin at the Rotunda Hospital. The conditions there were much the same as described by McCourt except that in Dublin, unlike Limerick, the slums were in what in the eighteenth century had been fine Georgian mansions.

By 1949 these great houses had fallen on hard times. Each of the main rooms now accommodated a different family serving not only as a bedroom but also as kitchen and living room. Each had a gas ring but the tap, which provided for the whole building and the toilet, shared by all, was at the bottom of the stairs in the yard. As far as health services were concerned, nothing at that time existed in Ireland to match the National Heath Service, which in the United Kingdom had just come into being in the previous year. There were, however, a number of famous hospitals supported by various charities and the Church, with not least at the Rotunda, clinical excellence and a long, proud tradition of teaching.

After a week's instruction in the elements of obstetrics in the delivery room at the Rotunda under the eye of a fearsome senior midwife, we students in teams of three – one of us with a bike as there were no reliable public telephones, went out 'on call' for deliveries in the district. Bearing in mind that few, if any of the mothers had received any antenatal care, we had to be prepared for anything. So first of all we had to learn by heart various rules of procedure. One, which has stuck in my mind to this day, was 'the list of indications for seeking immediate assistance'. Three of these: 'antepartum haemorrhage; prolapsed umbilical cord and epileptic fits due to eclampsia' remain indelibly engraved on my mind – although happily as it turned out, purely by luck, none of these nightmare complications arose in any of our patients.

The team to which I was assigned was unusual in that it consisted in addition to myself, of an ex-officer in the Coldstream Guards with a late vocation for medicine and a high caste Indian lady in a sari – the spectacular presence of the latter being regarded by our clientele as an infallible portent of good luck. And so it turned out to be.

Having taken our place on the rota and armed ourselves with *'Little's Practical Guide to Midwifery'*; some surgical gloves; a few simple instruments and a bar of soap, we settled down to wait for our turn of duty to come – the call for help usually arriving at the Rotunda in the shape of a more or less breathless relative on a bicycle.

However, all this led up to something of an anticlimax, for when with bated breath we arrived 'to conduct' our first delivery, we found that the mother, who had probably survived five or even ten deliveries, was the 'expert' and a deal less worried than we were. We, if the truth were known, were the beginners who needed her help, not the other way around.

It all sounds perilous now, and indeed seemed so to us at the time but in the event calamities rarely happened. What remains deeply engraved in my memory are the social conditions and the environment in which the deliveries took place – a social lesion with a vengeance. Little had altered since my father's time half a century before. The dilapidated room often had some of the Georgian plasterwork still intact. There was usually a coal fire burning in the grate which meant that in obstetrics sense, if push came to shove, chloroform (not ether which is explosive) had to be used. There was the huge bed occupying most of the room; barefoot children waiting on the stairs; father usually in the pub across the road; the cry of the mother as the baby was born; wads of newspaper to mop up the mess; the picture of the Holy Family on the wall; and, to add the final touch, being devoured by fleas.

Nowadays everything is different. But in those days, long before Ireland had any kind of 'welfare state'; and when in Dublin not only the termination of pregnancy but contraceptives of all kinds were unobtainable, our modest ministrations as students were not only acceptable but also welcomed. When the baby had arrived safely and had been swaddled there was often a cup of tea all round. As for us, we were growing up rapidly. But as if to confront us favoured young people with the consequences of the appalling poverty which surrounded us providence ordained that the first child we delivered was anencephalic – a horrific malformation of the brain incompatible with life. Anencephaly was at that time totally mysterious, but is now known to be due to a diet deficient in folic acid which is present in fresh vegetables, an item of food rarely found in the food of Dubliners in those days. Despite the dreadful deformity, having been solemnly enjoined that, whatever our personal beliefs, every baby at risk of death must be baptised immediately; we got some water, blessed it and to be on the safe side, gently gave the little girl the benefit.

As I reflect on my life, I grew up intellectually at that moment in Oxford when Percy O'Brien, having set me the topic of my first essay said "the ball's in your court, now." But as a middle-class lad from a privileged home, it was my experience of the Dublin slums and later of emergency admissions at the Middlesex, which put me in touch with social reality and made a man of me.

That reality sometimes assumed unexpected dimensions. Very recently at a formal dinner in London I was approached by a fellow guest I did not recognize. He was laughing,

"Do you remember the last time we met?" he asked. *"It was in Casualty at the Middlesex in 1953 and you were teaching me how to do a stomach wash out. I'm sure you'll remember!"*

He went on,

"The patient was an unconscious young woman who'd taken a huge overdose. As you said to me, "always listen to be sure the tube's in the stomach not the bronchus," and you held it to your ear, she vomited all over you. Your clothes were soaked from head to foot."

I did remember that incident from the distant past vividly, but for another reason! It brought back to my mind the sense of shock when, a few hours later, I discovered that my young patient had been pregnant and in trying to abort herself, had inflicted grievous damage to her body. A skilled surgeon saved her life but he told me it was doubtful whether she would conceive again.

The Great Smog of London 1952
One weekend in the winter of 1952 I happened to be in charge of emergency admissions at the Middlesex when an event occurred which the Registrar General's chief medical statistician was later to call 'a catastrophe of the first magnitude'. This was what is now remembered as 'the Great Smog of London'. 'Pea soupers', the jocular term by which Londoners in those days described the fogs which occurred regularly in the city each winter, were all too familiar to us. But both in density and duration, the Great Smog was of a different magnitude. It proved to be a turning point, which led to radical change.

Five days later when the dense toxic yellow vapour which had greeted Londoners as they drew back their curtains on Friday 5th December dispersed, more than 4,000 of them were dead. A public health tragedy had occurred only paralleled twice in the previous century – at the height of the cholera epidemic of 1854 - and in the global influenza epidemic of 1918-19.

My own personal memories of the Great Smog are vivid. The pall of fog, partly because it brought traffic almost to a standstill, also brought with it an eerie silence. It swirled about the streets and into the hospital wards so that the lights had to be switched on at midday, the smuts gradually turning the baths and washbasins deepening shades of grey. Although I had lived in the area for several years, I became completely disorientated when walking from Mortimer Street to Oxford Circus. It was only with great difficulty and by feeling my way along the walls of the buildings until I reached a street sign that I found my way back the few hundred yards to the Hospital.

Many people died at home without help. But others managed to reach us, the ambulance often having a guide walking in front, burning a flare to illuminate the curb.

By Saturday afternoon every spare bed in the Hospital was occupied by men and women, mostly elderly, gasping for breath. To make room I had to ask permission to cancel all routine admissions for the next week. But many people died in spite of everything we could do for them. Over the ensuing days, major problems also occurred in the disposal of the dead. The mortuaries and the Chapels of Rest were overwhelmed.

And what was the source of these lethal fumes? Not, as I believed at the time, London's factory chimneys. The cause was closer to home. What had effectively blacked out London in a toxic pall was the smoke of cheap coal[14] from two million grates trapped over the city in a 'cold snap' with no wind to blow it away. But good came from evil. The tragedy led on to the Clean Air Act of 1962 and eventually to the introduction of smokeless fuels.

---

[14] Cheap coal was in use because due to the War, Britain was almost bankrupt, and we were exporting our best coal to make ends meet.

CHAPTER 6
New Worlds

In the 1950s, as may still be the case today, it was usual for young British doctors, if they hoped, as I did, to end up in a teaching job at a University Hospital, to study for a period in the United States. And so it was that with financial help from a Travelling Fellowship of University College, Oxford, I found myself on a draughty day in December 1957 in Southampton boarding a passenger liner bound for America. Although it turned out to be an uneventful voyage in calm water, it has left me with vivid recollections. The first is of my companion in the double cabin which I had been allotted. He was a Dane whose internal clock seemed to have a setting which was the reciprocal of mine. Throughout the crossing we never saw enough of each other to hold a conversation. Each morning as I rolled out of my berth, he would stagger into the cabin, say "I am tronk" and collapse fully clothed on his bed. When I returned in the evenings he had gone.

My other memory of the voyage is more poignant. The liner called at Cobh, the deep-sea anchorage near Cork, to pick up Irish emigrants. I watched at the rail as a swarm of small boats packed with people came out to meet us, as we rode at anchor in the bay. Some came to sell shillelaghs and other trinkets but they were a minority. Amidst the sobs of relatives and the waving of scarves and handkerchiefs, a procession of men, women and children clutching parcels and bursting suitcases clambered up the gangway and disappeared into the ship. I have often wondered how many of these families were ever to see each other again.

My stay in America did not follow the orthodox pattern of the period. This would have involved study at one or other of the centres with world-wide acclaim, such as the Massachusetts General Hospital in Boston; Stanford in California or the Mayo Clinic. Instead I found myself first acting as Chief Resident in Medicine at a busy hospital in

Brooklyn, New York, and then on an attachment to the Charity Hospital in New Orleans, Louisiana. Finally I spent a year doing research in Washington, DC using the huge and at that time as yet still unexploited data bank of United States servicemen of the World Wars. All these experiences proved fascinating and the last in particular had an important influence on my career which more than forty years on continues to develop.

How an Ulster Protestant like myself came to be appointed Chief Resident in Medicine in an Orthodox Jewish hospital in Brooklyn is a mystery lost in the mists of time. But it cannot have been a coincidence that the only other Gentile in the hospital staff, who held the equivalent chief resident post in Surgery, was a Scot from Skye called McLeod. To make exceptions for appointments at this level obviously suited the hospital and it certainly suited me.

As the liner 'America' docked in New York, my new boss, Dr Max Michael, with the hospitality and friendliness which I was to learn is characteristic of the New World, was waiting for me on the pier on E.52nd Street. Having recently seen the film, 'Gone with the Wind', I knew as soon as he opened his mouth that he came from the Deep South. Max had been born and raised in Atlanta, Georgia. Together we loaded my luggage into his rather battered Dodge convertible. We then set off for his home where he put me up until I found an apartment.

But I remember Max Michael not so much as an excellent clinician who taught me a great deal but because of a conversation we had when I had got to know him well. I had asked him what he felt about the American Civil War. His expression changed.

"That was not a civil war," he said, *"it was a war between the States! We believed that except for foreign affairs,"* he went on, *"sovereignty rested not with Washington but with each State. If a State had a fundamental disagreement, it had the right to secede."*

"But surely it was right to abolish slavery?" I asked.
There was a pause.

"Maybe so," he replied, *"but hundreds of thousands died in that war. Anyway, in those days the Negroes in the South had jobs, shelter and plenty to eat. You should sure go see right here in Harlem how their great-grandchildren live today! Then make up your own mind. One day they'll burn the town down!"*

I never did dare to go see except from a taxi. But they did try to 'burn the town down', and later also tried to do the same in Washington and Los Angeles. In the years since the 'War between the States' with few exceptions at that time, freedom had brought them little more than poverty, poor housing and ill health. Looking back, the conversation I had with Max Michael in 1957 resonates with my much more recent experiences in Yugoslavia and the Chechnya region of Russia. Also with my upbringing in Belfast. A community divided by a 'social lesion' can be deceptively quiet for generations and then erupt over an apparently trivial incident. When Max Michael put his views to me almost a century had already elapsed since Gettysburg.

Although at the Maimonides Hospital almost all the staff were Jewish and the food in the doctor's dining room was kosher, the patients came from all the polyglot communities of Brooklyn. They included not only Italians, Jews, Irish and Puerto Ricans, but also

Greeks, Hungarians and Poles. Many of these were first generation immigrants who did not speak English. But one patient in particular who I can still see in my mind's eye was very far from being an immigrant. He was a tall, gaunt, rather sad-looking man who worked as a steel erector on the Manhattan skyscrapers and had high blood pressure. He turned out to be one of America's original inhabitants, an American Indian of the Iroquois tribe.

Although the variety of disease at the Maimonides differed from London, my task as chief resident was similar to the one I had fulfilled as a Resident Medical Officer at the Middlesex. At Maimonides I was responsible, as in London, for the day-to-day care of emergency cases and for overseeing the junior staff. When necessary I called for help from the 'attending' staff. These specialists, as had been the case in Britain before the NHS, were not paid for their services, but worked for the prestige of being associated with a University Hospital and for the contacts this fostered to the benefit of their private practices.

But there was one fundamental difference, which threw clinical practice in England into sharp contrast and affected my daily work. In Brooklyn, unless the person was completely destitute, the cost of everything – be it medicines, investigations or days in hospital, had to be met by the patient. Was the blood count, the barium meal, the scan, the biopsy really essential I constantly had to ask myself? In itself this was a prudent question which doctors should ask themselves more often wherever they practice. But in Brooklyn even when the answer was 'yes', there was a risk that some might go without for lack of funds. If I ever had any doubt about the importance of 'socialised medicine' as some Americans still refer disparagingly to the NHS, this was dispelled once and for all in Brooklyn.

"The British system will go bankrupt," said my American friends in 1958, *"it's only been going for ten years, you'll see."*

But they turned out to be wrong. More than fifty years on, the NHS is still there, in terms of financial support struggling as ever but nevertheless seemingly invincible.

In June 1959 I said goodbye to my friends in Brooklyn and set off to New Orleans in Louisiana on the next stage of my American adventure. My sojourn in New Orleans was the nearest I will ever get to living in the tropics. As the city is in the Mississippi delta the air not surprisingly is humid and in the afternoons when, as often happens, the temperature rises to the 90s, the heat becomes insufferable. As at that time I was hoping to specialise in diseases of the stomach and intestines, I had been recommended to work with a senior gastroenterologist in the city, Dr Gordon McHardy. Gordon divided his time between his own clinic where he saw his private patients and the Charity Hospital, a large institution in the city centre. In view of the climate and the fact that the hospital was not air-conditioned, we 'made rounds' with him starting at 7am. He was usually back in his comfortably cool clinic by 11 o'clock.

But in New Orleans there was also the fascination of seeing exotic diseases I had only read about in textbooks. Tularemia, which is the first cousin to bubonic plague (the Black Death), had smitten an unfortunate black woman who had punctured her hand on a bone whilst skinning a rabbit. Another woman, also a farm worker, had contracted an unpleasant fungal disease called blastomycosis. Up river in the Federal Leprosarium at Shreveport (now long since closed), I made a special trip to see the last American case of leprosy. I am glad to say all three patients recovered.

The Charity Hospital of New Orleans is run by nuns of the St Vincent de Paul order. In my time these statuesque ladies with their high hats and wimples provided the management of the hospital and oversaw the staff on the wards. The patients were segregated according to race – 'whites' in wards on one side of the hospital – which like the Middlesex was built in the form of a letter 'H' – and 'blacks' on the other. The financial arrangements were similar to those at the Middlesex prior to the NHS. The patients, none of whom had health insurance, and all of whom came from the poorer sectors of the community were assessed by a social worker to determine what contribution they could make.

Shortly before I left Louisiana, the legislation which made racial segregation unlawful, came into force. Next day I looked with interest to see what would happen. Although the notices saying 'Whites' and 'Blacks' had been removed little else had changed. In the bus, which took me to work, the moveable boards across the gangway, which divided the seating by race, had also gone. But whites still sat at the front and blacks at the back in their accustomed places. Change involving more than lip service was going to take time. This was not surprising, as segregation had divided New Orleans society since the arrival of the first settlers and their slaves in the seventeenth century.

A few years later, by a quirk of fate I happened to be in South Africa when a step in precisely the opposite direction took place and the 'apartheid' laws came into force. I was visiting the Groote Schuur Hospital in Capetown and was sitting in the office of a senior doctor which looked out immediately above the main entrance. He broke off our discussion and pointed to the taxi rank outside.

"You see those taxis?" he said, *"That rank has been there since time immemorial and serves everyone. By custom the drivers have always been Indians. From tomorrow they will all be out of a job. The new 'apartheid' law will mean that they cannot take whites or blacks as passengers – each race will have to provide its own taxis."*

And as he went on with indignation,

"You are a witness to a rich and beautiful country committing suicide!"

And so it turned out to be. From that day on, until the election of the Mandela government twenty years later, South Africa was isolated and deprived not only of most of its markets but of all its other international activities, including its tourist industry and sport.

A Goldmine in Washington

As I look back on my career, my second year in the United States proved to be a turning point. The path I then followed gradually led me away from clinical practice to the wider field of public health. On leaving the Charity Hospital at New Orleans my next place of study, the Office of the US Veterans Administration in Washington, was chosen because I believed its huge archive of records of literally millions of ex-servicemen from all over the North American continent, might contain clues about the origins of disease. I turned out to be correct.

But first of all there was an amusing formality. As a British citizen, how was I to gain access to what were in legal terms confidential records belonging to the US Government? The archives could only be opened to a 'United States Marshal' – a term I had previously only heard of in the context of 'Wild West' films about cowboys and Indians. The solution to the problem was obvious. Having first made discreet enquiries at the British Embassy that I would not thereby lose my citizenship, I was duly sworn in before a magistrate. For all I know, I continue to this day to be a Federal Marshal of the United States of America.

The files of the VA Central Office in Washington turned out to be an epidemiological goldmine, which, in terms of scale, can have few rivals worldwide. However, their unique value lies in the way in which by 'record linkage' they accumulate the histories of each person over a lifetime.

Could events or experiences in early life, recorded when the person was examined for entry to the U.S. Forces, I wondered, cast light on the causes or severity of later illnesses?

To a relative novice like myself, an important bonus was the presence in the VA Central Office of a number of distinguished scientists. These included Gilbert Beebe's team who were working on the long-term effects on the Japanese population of the atomic bombs dropped on Hiroshima and Nagasaki in 1945, and Clifford Bachrach, the statistician. Contact with these scientists on an almost daily basis over the next twelve months gave me my grounding in epidemiology and statistics.

But how should I focus my work? I only had a year to spare and the opportunities offered were almost infinite. As my career plan at that time was to follow one of my mentors at the Middlesex and train as a specialist in the diseases of the stomach and intestines, should I concentrate on these? On the other hand, I was still fascinated by what I had learned from Douglas McAlpine about multiple sclerosis (MS) and its strange global distribution. Might the pattern of this disease of the central nervous system among U.S. ex-servicemen recruited from all over America, provide a clue to its cause? My interest in MS was reinforced by the fact that my cousin David was severely disabled by it and that he had been given the somewhat impractical and as we now know inappropriate advice to emigrate to South Africa where, he was correctly told, the disease did not occur in people of British and Dutch extraction born there.

In the end I managed to cram in some work on both of these topics. When I look back, although my achievements in intestinal diseases were modest, they have stood the test of time and edged the frontiers of knowledge forward a little. As for my work on multiple sclerosis, fifty years later it is leading on to greater things.

From among the diseases of the bowel I chose two which although not particularly common, often result in serious and sustained ill health. Ulcerative colitis and regional enteritis cause inflammation respectively of the colon and small intestine together with troublesome diarrhoea. My contribution was to draw attention to features which perhaps point to a common genetic factor underlying their origin. Thus I found that men of Jewish origin suffered from these diseases at least twice as often as do people of other ethnic backgrounds. Also that each may occur at different times in the same person and that both may be complicated by a rare stiffening form of arthritis of the spine, 'bamboo spine', or to give its official name 'ankylosing spondylitis'. Although these points were of some academic interest, they have sadly not led to advances which have been of any benefit to patients.

Of more practical importance was my finding that some people who have suffered from ulcerative colitis are at risk later of developing cancer in the inflamed area of the bowel. By pointing to the patterns of disease which predispose to cancer, this work may have encouraged vigilance and early diagnosis, in time for curative surgical treatment to be carried out.

But in retrospect, my work on the paralytic diseases of the brain and spinal cord 'multiple sclerosis' (MS) in veterans has proved more important. Indeed, looking back at it almost half a century later, it seems that I have stumbled on a significant clue to the cause of this tragic illness.

Does lack of sunshine cause multiple sclerosis?

My starting point was the acknowledged fact that among susceptible people such as those of British and North European stock, there are major unexplained geographic variations in incidence in different parts of the world. Thus in South Africa and the sub tropical Australian state of Queensland, the European settlers rarely develop MS, while in New Zealand, the disease is common. This strongly suggests that the key to the cause of the disease must be in the environment. Does this pattern reflect differences in climate acting <u>directly</u>, as I wrote "by the operation of cold, heat or sunshine on the human body", or <u>indirectly</u> by the effect of climate on diet or lifestyle? I wondered whether a detailed study of MS in United States ex-servicemen who had been recruited from all parts of a continent which has major variations in climate would help clarify the issue.

And so it turned out to be! The pattern of birthplace of veterans who developed MS after they joined the US Armed Forces differed significantly from other veterans. More of those with MS came from the north and fewer from the south than expected from the general pattern of recruitment. This gradient seemed consistent at all longitudes of the continent from west to east. Was there a clue to the cause of MS in this pattern?

Further work showed that veterans who had spent their early life in parts of the United States with a sunny climate – perhaps particularly in winter – were least likely to develop MS. The statistics suggested that the amount of sunshine rather than the absence of cold weather in the climate might be the protective factor. Could exposure to sunshine really protect people from developing MS? It seemed surprising to say the least, even far-fetched and when I mentioned it to colleagues, I was met with incredulity even ridicule.

A fearsome example of this occurred when after my return I spoke about it by invitation to an elite audience at the National Hospital for Nervous Diseases, Queen Square: *"Sunshine prevent MS?"* said Sir Francis Walshe who as the doyen of British Neurology was chairing the meeting, *"What absolute poppycock, dear boy; moonshine you mean, complete moonshine!"*

From this experience two things became obvious. If I were to be taken seriously I would need more data; and a career in clinical neurology was not for me.

Fortunately, while my colleagues and I were working in the northern hemisphere parallel work was taking place in the southern hemisphere, the key investigator being John Sutherland, a British neurologist who had settled in Queensland. As a Scot, Sutherland had been surprised by the virtual absence of cases of MS in Brisbane, where he now practiced, compared with his native Glasgow where it was among the commonest diseases he encountered.

My next contribution was to take John Sutherland's work a step further and, using mortality rates as an indicator, to look at all the European settler populations in the Southern Hemisphere – Australia, New Zealand and South Africa. It turned out that in the Southern Hemisphere there was also a gradient in the prevalence of MS from south to north, exactly as one would predict if sunshine in early life protected susceptible people from developing the disease. In Australia, the highest rate was in Tasmania, the lowest in Western Australia and Queensland; likewise in New Zealand, MS is commoner in the South rather than the North island; while in South Africa, MS is almost unknown other than in immigrants who have spent their youth in Europe.

More than forty years ago when there appeared to be no credible mechanism whereby such an effect could occur, I was cautious about drawing the obvious conclusion. This is that solar radiation – presumably through the action of ultraviolet light on the skin – can protect susceptible people from developing MS. Two contemporary studies within the continent of Australia further reinforce this point. The first shows that the negative correlation between exposure to ultraviolet light (UVL) and the prevalence of MS is even closer than the positive relationship with the incidence of malignant melanoma, furthermore the equation for the regression line between the prevalence of multiple sclerosis and ultra violet light is identical in both Northern and Southern hemispheres. This rules out any possibility that the relationship is due to a confounding factor. The second and the more important of the two, as it deals with individuals rather than geographical patterns has found that in Tasmania, where the disease is relatively common, sunbathing in early life protects against MS. A final point which in my view fills the 'bucket of certainty' to overflowing, has emerged by remarkable coincidence from work based on data from the Oxford Record Linkage Study. In Britain, skin cancer develops less commonly in people with MS than in those with other autoimmune diseases. So even in cloudy Britain it seems that exposure to sunshine can protect people from multiple sclerosis.

Recent work approaching this problem from an entirely different direction has provided an important new clue. Unlikely as it may seem, this comes from work on rodents. Laboratory experiments have shown that a disease resembling multiple sclerosis in rats may be prevented by injections of Vitamin D – a substance present in the diet but which, in humans, is also synthesised by the action of UVL on the skin. As might be expected this finding was rapidly followed by attempts to help patients with MS, treating them with Vitamin D. The fact that so far this has proved unsuccessful by no means eliminates what is now a likelihood, that sunshine acting via Vitamin D or one of its derivatives may indeed protect people from developing MS.

Although fifty years on I am now certain that exposure to sunshine in early life protects against the development of MS, it is frustrating that this suggestion has so far proved of such little benefit to patients. What remains clear however, is that if a British family decides to emigrate to South Africa, Queensland, Western Australia or to California, the risk of their children developing MS will be remote, while elsewhere in the English-speaking world, for example, in Canada, the Northern States of the USA and New Zealand, there will be a significant risk of the disease.

A Bitter Disappointment

My stay in the United States ended with a disappointment which at the time seemed devastating. But like the ending of a fairy tale, it eventually turned out to be a blessing in disguise. The bad news arrived in a letter from Sir Francis Avery Jones, at that time doyen of British gastroenterology who had promised to sponsor me on my return to England. The message was plain to the point of rudeness. He had found someone else to fill the post he had promised me. He therefore would not after all require my services. I thought of the injunction in scripture: *"Put not your trust in princes!"* and for some weeks remained in a state of shock. Should I try for US citizenship and remain in Washington? Should I emigrate to Australia or New Zealand? Then, as it seemed completely out of the blue, but in fact perhaps because my research was now beginning to appear in scientific journals read in Britain, came another letter, this time post-marked Oxford.

Although I could not have predicted it at the time, this letter led on to a series of opportunities which even today, forty years later, has not run its full course. It also had a more immediate and agreeable consequence. The closure of the road to gastroenterology meant that I would be spared the fate of spending a significant part of my life performing 'endoscopy', in other words, poking flexible telescopes from below to search for signs of disease in the rectum or from above to look for ulcers in the stomach. Patients also benefited because to do these investigations properly requires a degree of manual dexterity I simply do not possess.

CHAPTER 7
Back to Oxford

The second letter, which sometime in the autumn of 1959 found its way into the mailbox of my house on the outskirts of Washington, came from Leslie Witts, at that time Professor of Medicine at Oxford. Witts' department was one of several recently financed by a gift from the motor car tycoon William Morris, later to be known as Lord Nuffield, Britain's equivalent to Henry Ford. I accepted Witts' invitation to join him not only with profound relief but with enthusiasm. At that time, the Nuffield Department of Medicine was at the peak of its reputation and was attracting post-graduate students from all over the world.

Leslie Witts was an unusual man. Not only was he one of the few clinicians outside the realm of psychiatry who had himself undergone psychoanalysis but he espoused the then controversial principles of what was known as 'social medicine'. These included the obvious but at the time seemingly revolutionary view that physical illness was often due to social or psychological factors.

But there was far more to this shy and retiring man than met the eye. He had the rare gift of creating an atmosphere in his department where not only was good work done and new ideas were discussed, but there was little sense of hierarchy. This meant that young doctors like myself were given space to grow in confidence and stature. It was at one of the weekly clinical conferences when patients whose symptoms were proving difficult to treat were discussed, that an unforgettable event took place.

The patient, a young woman with many symptoms who was steadily losing weight, had been passed unavailingly from doctor to doctor and had undergone every conceivable type of test and investigation. As no underlying cause had been found, doctors, friends, and family alike were becoming increasingly anxious and alarmed. Witts looked through the clinical notes; smiled at the patient; asked her one or two general questions, and gently invited her to go back to the ward. Then came the bombshell.

"I am disappointed that none of you has thought to enquire whether this young woman has achieved satisfaction in her sexual relationship", said Witts. *"After all, her notes show that the symptoms began almost exactly at the time of her marriage last year."*

In 1960, twenty-five years before AIDS, and when precious little sex education took place in schools – or indeed anywhere else – this comment was a sensation. As it turned out, Witts proved to be correct. With appropriate specialist help we soon had not only a grateful patient but also a much happier couple. Later, when I became Dean of the new medical school at Southampton, I made sure that 'Human Reproduction' including sexology, had a prominent place at the beginning of the course. While I cannot prove this course was effective, it was certainly popular, which in teaching is more than half the battle.

Working with Witts, but of a totally different temperament, was an equally distinguished physician whose encouragement also proved to have a profound influence on my career. Sidney Truelove's contribution, which was a singular one, was to the science of treatment or 'therapeutics' to give it its full name. Up to that time, unbelievable as it may seem today, new drugs tended to be introduced on a simple trial and error 'let's try it out on a few people and see if it works' basis, a method which often led to misleading and occasionally to disastrous results.

Sidney was a pioneer of the 'randomised controlled trial' without which today it would be unthinkable – indeed unlawful – for a new treatment to be introduced. In simple terms, by this method half a group of patients with a particular disease are allocated at random to the best treatment currently available, while the other half receive the new treatment. In such trials, not only must all of the patients have given informed consent, but also today the proposal must have been agreed by an independent ethical committee. In my time, at one level I saw Sidney's trials lead to significant advances in the treatment of ulcerative colitis and other conditions in which the Department specialised but at another I found myself as an onlooker sharing in the excitement of witnessing the first examples of what has unquestionably turned out to have been the most important advance in therapeutics of the 20th century.

But it was in a different area that Sidney's influence was to prove crucial to the development of my own career. It turned out that his own experience as a doctor in the Royal Army Medical Corps in Italy in the World War had convinced him of the importance of routine medical records for research. He was therefore not in the least surprised about my discoveries in Washington. In Italy, a simple analysis of records had revealed that two different epidemics of jaundice were happening among the troops at the same time not one. Cases of hepatitis due to drinking infected water with an incubation period of thirty days were occurring alongside cases of syringe borne jaundice with an incubation period of ninety days – the latter having originated from faulty sterilisation of equipment used for giving the soldiers injections. This analysis had led swiftly to appropriate action and control of both epidemics.

It was against this background that in 1961[15] Sidney Truelove and I, together with Leslie Witts jointly submitted a letter entitled 'National Epidemiology' to the British Medical Journal which led in due course to the setting up of the Oxford Record Linkage Study (ORLS). We envisaged that such a system should it eventually become national "would make it possible to follow the medical record of an individual from the cradle to the grave", "create a science of prognosis" and within a few years "provide valuable material about childhood diseases, e.g. acute leukaemia." The letter was welcomed with enthusiasm by, amongst others, the psychiatrist Sir Aubrey Lewis, and Sir Richard Doll, the epidemiologist who had discovered the link between smoking and lung cancer.

In view of the favourable comment which ensured, we were able to recruit the enthusiastic support of the Chief Medical Officer, Sir George Godber who helped us in our search for financial support.

The outcome was that the Nuffield Trust funded a pilot study which set us four tasks:

1.   To find out if it was feasible to accumulate data about important health events from different sources – such as birth, admission to hospital and death for a defined population

2.   To develop computer methods to link the records into cumulative personal files

3.   To exploit the files as a tool for medical research

4.   If successful to promote extension of the system to a national scale

By the time I left Oxford in 1968, to become Dean of the new Medical School at Southampton, in partnership with my Australian colleague Michael Hobbs, we had made significant progress in achieving the first

---

[15] BMJ 1961 1 p668.

three objectives. We had also extended our coverage and the study was collecting key health records of a population of some 750,000 men, women and children.

Thirty-four years later the present Director, Professor Michael Goldacre, has just accepted the Government's invitation to extend the study to cover the whole of England. This achieves the fourth and last of the original tasks set by the Nuffield Trust forty years ago. This will also realise the prophetic vision of the great nineteenth century statistician William Farr who in 1875 in his 35th Report to the Registrar General envisaged a similar system which

"will tend to an invaluable contribution to therapeutics as well as to public health for it will enable physicians to determine the duration and fatality of all forms of disease under various treatments and social conditions of the people… the national returns of cases and causes of death will be an arsenal which the genius of English healers cannot fail to take into account."

Associations between diseases

My work in the USA had shown that the occurrence of two or more diseases at different times in the lifespan of a person may sometimes provide clues about the cause of the conditions or may help guide the clinician towards better treatment. Thus the way ulcerative colitis, Crohn's Disease and ankylosing spondylitis tended to occur together in the same patient suggested a common genetic factor, while the link of a risk of a subsequent cancer of the bowel among people who suffer from ulcerative colitis should have increased the vigilance of those patients' doctors. But if these associations had been discovered in a single year's study of the subsequent records of fit young Americans called up for military service, how much more might be discovered in the study of a population of men, women and children of all ages?

In the forty years which have now elapsed since the formation of the Oxford Record Linkage Study, in addition to confirming some well known links such as that between gastric ulcer and subsequent gastric cancer, the linked files have uncovered many previously unknown associations with an ever widening range of implications.

Some of the new discoveries are important because they provide reassurance. Thus men who have undergone the common sterilisation operation vasectomy will be relieved to know that no support has been found for the suspicion that this procedure might increase the risk of cancer of the testicle or prostate; likewise there is no support for the idea that removal of the gall bladder (cholecystectomy) predispose to bowel cancer.

Other links have been discovered which lead in a different direction. This is to help clarify the chain of events which lead to the occurrence of a disease. Thus the evidence that smoking in some mysterious way protects people from developing Parkinson's Disease fits in with the finding that lung cancer is significantly less common in people suffering from that condition. As yet equally mysterious is the fact that thyroid disease occurs more frequently than expected in people who suffer from asthma, but again there may be a clue here which in the future will prove useful.

But perhaps the most mysterious association which has so far been revealed by record linkage is the relationship between two important but very different diseases – schizophrenia and rheumatoid arthritis. The association is negative, in other words is in fact a <u>disassociation</u>. Thus only about half the expected number of cases of rheumatoid arthritis are found among schizophrenic patients. Yet there is no such negative relationship between rheumatoid arthritis and other types of psychiatric illness. Equally mysterious but more perplexing is the emerging evidence that termination of a pregnancy may be associated with an increased risk of breast cancer in later life.

Some of the associations between diseases that record linkage has uncovered have immediate clinical implications, many but not all of which are reassuring. In other instances the importance of the newly discovered relationship lies in its potential to stimulate a novel train of thought or a new line of research into unsolved problems of cause and effect.

So far, the associations mentioned relate to illnesses occurring at different times in the same person. If the records of mothers are linked with those of their children, a different perspective emerges with the possibility that clues in the maternal record may cast light on some of the health problems of infants and children. I conclude with two examples where, although the conditions are uncommon, it is important that doctors and nurses working with newborn babies should have them in mind.

Family record linkage
Cryptorchidism – failure of the descent of the testicles into the scrotum prior to birth – affects approximately 1% of boys and is a serious condition associated not only with infertility but with a subsequent risk of cancer of the testicle. As the ORLS has linked mother-baby files for almost 1,500 boys with cryptorchidism, it has been possible to provide some vivid insights into why this anomaly happens. It turns out that it occurs particularly in boys whose mothers have suffered deprivation in pregnancy which has caused impaired placental function and foetal

growth. The consequence of maternal deprivation being not only failure of the testicles to descend but, even worse to an increased risk of diabetes in childhood. Fortunately along with this unhappy picture goes the hope that the finding may spur on greater efforts to encourage deprived women to seek early antenatal care to reduce these risks.

Congenital inguinal[16] hernia is a related condition. This is important to recognise for a different reason: because unless it is treated promptly it may strangulate and prove fatal. While inguinal hernia is about eight times more common in boys than girls, due to the monumental scale of the linked files, the Oxford Record Linkage Study has been able to make an important contribution to the care of girls with this type of hernia – of which it has identified so far no fewer than 2,534 cases – and in particular to the sisters of these girls who are also potentially at risk. Basically the practical point which emerges is that not only the brothers but the sisters of children with inguinal hernia should be examined carefully at birth for this condition so that it can be treated before serious and sometimes fatal complications develop.

Record Linkage in the Antipodes

It is no coincidence that Howard Newcombe's idea that the study of health records collected over a lifetime might reveal previously undisclosed secrets is now flourishing in Australia. The reason for this is that Michael Hobbs who in the 1960's was my principal colleague in the development of the Oxford Record Linkage Study is an Australian. On his return to Perth in 1967, Michael pioneered a system of linked records covering the whole of Western Australia. Over the years a rich harvest has emerged from this work.

---

[16] A hernia, 'rupture', which occurs in the groin.

Two recent studies in particular show how record linkage techniques can lead to the discovery of totally new and unexpected clues to disease causation – in this case the very different but devastating conditions – cancer and congenital malformations, both of which are difficult to prevent and cure.

Briefly, the Western Australian studies have shown that cancer of the prostate is three times more common among men who are allergic to house mite infested dust than others;® and that babies conceived by <u>in vitro</u> fertilisation have about double the risk of certain congenital malformations than those normally conceived.®

In Western Australia record linkage is currently also being used as a tool in a variety of studies in the more mundane but nevertheless important area of quality care within the health and social services.®

Recently New Zealand has also begun to employ record linkage. The technique is being used in analyses of the quality of primary healthcare and in unravelling the causes of coronary heart disease.

Record linkage comes of age

From the time of the early population Censuses, people in Britain have felt strongly that data which they have provided for statistical purposes should be treated as strictly confidential. When one considers that in 1962 when the Oxford Record Linkage Study (ORLS) was founded, the appalling abuses by Nazi Germany of personal data banks was still fresh in people's minds, I think I was fortunate even with the support of the Chief Medical Officer of those days, Sir George Godber, to have got agreement to set the study up. More recently Britain's entry into the European Community set even stricter criteria for the security of personal data and the Data Protection Agency was created as a public watchdog. All this being so, the recent invitation by the Government to Professor Michael Goldacre, the ORLS' current Director, to extend the study to cover the whole of England is remarkable. It is both at long last an acknowledgement of the importance of linked data as a research tool and a tribute to the study's unblemished reputation for security.

But the success of the Oxford Record Linkage Study has also encouraged others to follow. Among the most remarkable developments of record linkage have been within the government's Office of National Statistics in London. These have included the creation in the 1980s of a Longitudinal Study in which information about health and social status are linked throughout the lifespan for a 1% sample of the population; an Infant and Childhood File which links information about parents to social and biological data about pregnancy, infancy and childhood; and a Cancer Study which deals with the causes and treatment of malignant disease.

These linked files have already yielded a rich harvest of results with important implications. Not only has record linkage shown that poverty in childhood may shorten life but that so also may unemployment. These findings have led to urgent changes in policy including the 'Sure Start' initiative targeting support to children in need, and the relegation to the dust heap of policies which used the deliberate creation of unemployment as a regulator of the economy. The Longitudinal Study has produced another surprise. This is that poor health in deprived neighbourhoods is more likely to be improved by targeting individuals who live in them rather than by attending to the environmental deficiencies of the locality.

Although the Infant and Childhood Linked Mortality files have also provided valuable information with an impact on maternity services and on the government's policies on teenage pregnancy, it is the <u>Cancer</u> file which has had the greater impact. This, with humiliating clarity, has spotlighted serious deficiencies in Britain's cancer services. Not only does the success of treatment vary unacceptably from place to place but in many areas results are significantly worse than in other comparable countries abroad. Thereby record linkage has shattered a deep-seated area of complacency and in so doing will eventually provide a sound basis for improvements.

As a technique, record linkage can properly be considered as having outgrown its controversial beginnings and should now be accepted as an established and valuable tool for the furtherance of sound social policies and effective healthcare.

The nasal cancer study

But something else happened while I was in Oxford which shows how important it is for people working in public health to keep in touch with clinicians. One day at lunch in the doctor's dining room at the Radcliffe Infirmary, I happened to sit down opposite Ronald Macbeth and Esmé Hadfield, the senior consultants in ear, nose and throat surgery. Theirs was a highly specialised field with which I had had little contact since my student days.

"You're interested in epidemics, aren't you?"

said Ronald Macbeth, taking his eye for a moment off his plate of cottage pie and adjusting his spectacles. At this point I remember wondering what on earth would happen next. Had there been an outbreak of infection in the operating theatre?

"Well, I'm beginning to wonder whether, in our work, my colleague Esmé Hadfield and I have seen an epidemic evolving before our very eyes!"

In the next few minutes a story emerged which, in the end, led not only to the discovery of what is now known as the 'furniture makers' cancer, an otherwise extremely rare tumour of the inner lining of the nose and an industrial hazard subsequently found in many other countries throughout the world, but to a similar hazard in a seemingly unrelated industry as well.

Ronald Macbeth told me that over the years, a steady flow of patients with this tumour had been referred to him and his colleague from High Wycombe for treatment – all without exception having worked in one or other of the town's furniture factories. Would I like to do an investigation? I accepted with enthusiasm, and the project, which we conducted jointly, turned out to be one of the most interesting of my career.

When we got down to work it soon became clear that the cancers which Ronald and Esmé had originally thought were due to the inhalation of chemicals in the stains and varnishes applied to the finished chairs and tables in fact occurred in a different part of the factory. They developed exclusively in men exposed to the dust generated earlier in the process. This dust arises when the timber is sawn up, turned and sanded before the parts are assembled while as might be expected staining and varnishing can only take place in a dust free environment. Further, as the tumours did not appear until at least twenty-five years after the men had started work, it was Chiltern beech familiar to all of us in Britain, which must have been the culprit not the more recently imported exotic timbers from the tropics. Who could have dreamt for a moment that beeches, those beautiful trees with trunks extending to a hundred feet, silver-blue bark and spreading shade, could possibly cause cancer? But the truth is that in their sawdust there is indeed a carcinogen concealed! Subsequently the furniture makers' cancer has been identified in a number of other countries using similar timber, including the Netherlands and Denmark.

But the story does not end there. With the help of the local cancer registry, we were able to map the cases of nasal cancer occurring in other parts of the Oxford region. As expected, there was a major cluster in High Wycombe associated with its chair making industry, with a smaller focus of patients in Banbury – although we had not realised it – who we later discovered also had a furniture factory. But why were there also cases in Northamptonshire where we could find no evidence that a furniture industry ever existed? Could this rare cancer also be a problem among the workers in Northamptonshire's famous boot and shoe industry?

Further study gave the answer. Nasal cancer does indeed occur among shoemakers but is limited to those workers (a small minority) exposed to dust from the specially hardened leather used for soles and heels. This dust occurs as high speed grinding machines trim and shape the soles and heels before the shoes are assembled and also during repairs. Is there a biochemical link between the shoemakers' and furniture makers' cancers? Possibly. Although it has not been proved, it may be that tannins, contained in the liquid in which the leather for heels and soles is soaked to harden it and which are derived from extracts of the bark of trees may be the common factor.

There has also been a practical outcome to the work. In both industries the dust has been listed as potentially carcinogenic, proper ventilation has been installed and those affected compensated.

While I was in Oxford another event occurred in an entirely different aspect of my work which at the time some of my friends predicted would put an end to my career. I fell out publicly with one of the most influential doctors in the country – the President of the Royal College of Physicians, at that time, an irascible gentleman called Sir Robert Platt.

It happened like this. As well as research and clinical work, my job as Clinical Tutor in the Medical School included responsibility for organising the training of young doctors at Oxford aspiring to become specialist physicians. An essential stepping-stone was first to pass the examination entitling them to become members of the Royal College of Physicians of London. For British students, this was important enough as without the initials 'MRCP' after their names, there was little hope of progress up the promotion ladder. But for those from many parts of the Commonwealth where there was no equivalent to the National Health Service, it was absolutely indispensable. Without having first passed the MRCP examination, these doctors would have no credibility to earn their living as specialists.

As for the examination itself, it was in those days a disaster. There was no published curriculum of its requirements and no acknowledged course of instruction to prepare for it. Even good local candidates who had been lucky enough to train at teaching hospitals in Britain commonly failed the examination once or twice, while foreign students might try and fail five, ten or even twenty times. Yet the fees for candidates were high.

Early in 1963 two of my students – both conscientious and able people – failed the examination for the umpteenth time. My frustration boiled over and I wrote a sharp letter for publication in the British Medical Journal. This, which fortunately for me was supported in the same issue by a powerful leading article from the Editor not only expressed my concern about the fairness of the exam but went a long step further. It hinted that the Royal College's policy on the MRCP examination, if not actually guided by financial considerations, was probably influenced by them.

All hell broke loose. The President of the Royal College lost his temper and after he had left angry telephone messages at my home and elsewhere, a sharp rebuke from him appeared in the Press. In contrast my own mailbag was without exception favourable and occasionally funny. I remember two letters in particular. One from my father linked praise for supporting a good cause with hopes that, in future, I would try to avoid 'making enemies in high places'. Another came from a friend who impishly congratulated me on my 'Life Membership', in other words, hinting that after this public contretemps with the President, I could never expect election to the College's highest echelon – the Fellowship – but would remain permanently a 'Member'. Happily, events turned out otherwise. Time passed; the next President was elected; Sir Robert decamped to the House of Lords; and the Membership examination whether coincidentally or not was radically reformed roughly along the lines I had suggested. Shortly before my fortieth birthday, if anything a little earlier than was usual in those days, I was elected FRCP.

A Visit to the Holy Land

Sometime in 1966 I was invited by Sam Cohen, a colleague whose research was in the same field as mine, to an international conference in Israel on the use of computers in medicine. Unfortunately in the interim the 'Six Day War' between the Israelis and the Palestinians erupted and the conference was cancelled. But I need not have been disappointed for this turn of events led to one of the more memorable episodes in my life. Calm, if not peace, having been restored in Palestine within a few days, I decided I might as well use my plane ticket. I therefore phoned Sam Cohen and set off for Tel Aviv.

I remember little of my flight except that the plane was empty as indeed was the airport. I hailed a taxi and this brought my first surprise. An unmistakably Cockney voice answered.

"Jerusalem? My pleasure gov'ner!" You're the first fare I've had all day," and then *"There it is! Look!"* He pointed. *"Ain't it beautiful?"*

And so indeed it was. It's walls and towers unmistakable, gleaming in the sunshine along the ridge far above us. As for the road, we swung back and forth round seemingly an endless series of bends to an altitude equivalent to the top of Snowdon.

I do not remember where in the suburbs I stayed the first night. But I will never forget Sam Cohen's rejoinder when I phoned to say I had arrived.

"Wonderful, let's go together tomorrow to the Holy City. Do you realise that although I was born and raised here more than twenty-five years ago, I have never until now been allowed to cross the checkpoint at the Damascus Gate? This will be my very first visit."

At this point a word of explanation of the political situation is needed. Prior to the Six Day War, the partition of Palestine had been such that while the Jewish settlers had access to much of what is now known as Israel, including the extensive modern suburbs of Jerusalem, they were denied access to the Holy City itself which within its medieval walls had sites sacred not only to Christians and Moslems but also as might be expected, to Jews.

But now all that had changed. For the first time since the end of the UN Mandate in 1948 Jerusalem was open to all religions. Although more than thirty years have passed, my memories of what happened next are vivid. As, literally within a week of the end of the war, Jacob and I walked together through the Damascus Gate I wondered how often since the Crusades the Holy City had been so completely empty not only of tourists but of pilgrims.

The first sight that met our eyes was a surprise! An ancient Church propped and shored up by rusty scaffolding with the sound of chanting coming from within. While Sam stood respectfully outside, a Franciscan explained to me that this was none other than the Church of the Holy Sepulchre built on the site of Christ's burial. As all the ancient sects of Christianity had equal rights of access but bitter differences in belief and almost everything else, no agreement on upkeep had been reached in human memory. It therefore had fallen into disrepair and it had been left to the British Government, the secular occupying power, to do the minimum necessary to prevent the collapse of the building.

After that I remember a narrow curved street – the Way of the Cross – up which we were walking in the reverse direction to Jesus. It was almost deserted. A few shopkeepers were at their doors; some nuns; the pool of Silaom where the blind man washed his eyes and was cured. Then we reached the top. There was the Dome of the Rock with its mosque gleaming in the sunlight, and the 'Wailing Wall', the surviving fragment of Solomon's temple. An elderly Jew had his eyes fixed on it and swayed gently back and forward on his heels. But then there was an almost obscene anticlimax. On the right, its ammunition neatly stacked beside it and its muzzle poking through an embrasure, stood an unattended British Army 25 pounder field gun, a relic of the city's occupation until a few days ago by the Arab Legion.

Next day, having parted from my friend and spent the night in a hotel, I made enquiries about visiting Bethlehem which I knew was nearby.

"Impossible", said my hosts, *"all public transport is suspended."*
"But could I not walk?" I asked, *"It's only five miles."*

It turned out that this was indeed a possibility as there had been no fighting on the road. But I would be on my own. In those days I was too young and inexperienced to worry about such things as mines, or snipers.

And so it was that with my pack on my back I set off from the Holy City for Bethlehem. The suburbs of Jerusalem did not extend far in this direction and I was soon walking in open country. On either side, the landscape was seemingly as it had been for centuries, rocky with sparse grazing, sheep and goats and an occasional shepherd. I find that the road itself is indeed deserted.

After about an hour's walk there emerges a cluster of white buildings and towers. In Manger Square I am welcomed as a phenomenon by a small crowd who claim that they have seen no-one walking from this direction for several weeks. Competition to offer me a coffee – everyone speaking in English. Competition also from the custodians of the two entrances to the subterranean grotto where tradition claims Christ was born. Would the evident commercialisation and vulgarity with trinkets and hawkers destroy any sense of holiness? Not so. Again the lack of crowds comes to my aid. In a tiny alcove underground where lamps burn I kneel alone but for a Franciscan brother.

Having returned safely to Jerusalem by taxi, I set out for home.

Goodbye to Oxford

Sometime in 1967 when I had begun to think I would spend the rest of my life under the spell of Oxford and its University, two letters came through my post box which led to a turning point in my career. Both were marked 'Private'. The first I opened was from the Principal of my College (Brasenose), offering me a Professorial Fellowship. This was a rare and prestigious honour which would give me the security to develop the research potential of the ORLS and which no one in his right senses would dream of refusing. But as I was trying to absorb this welcome surprise, I opened the second letter. This put before me an entirely different opportunity in an unexpected field. In it was an invitation to become the first Dean of a new Medical School planned for Southampton. As so far there were neither students, detailed plans nor buildings, this would provide the first opportunity for innovation in medical education for more than fifty years.

Today with hindsight it seems obvious that the decision I eventually took was the right one but at the time this seemed much less clear. Unfortunately my prevarication and shilly-shallying was to lead to serious embarrassment. Thus some weeks later on successive days reports appeared in the press that I had been appointed to two different and incompatible jobs – the one in Oxford which in the end I turned down and the other in Southampton which I had just accepted.

Many years were to pass before Oxford forgave me. But in 1988 when I was Chief Medical Officer of England, another letter arrived with the Oxford postmark. This time it contained an invitation from the Principal of Brasenose that I should become an Honorary Life Fellow of the College. The world had moved on.

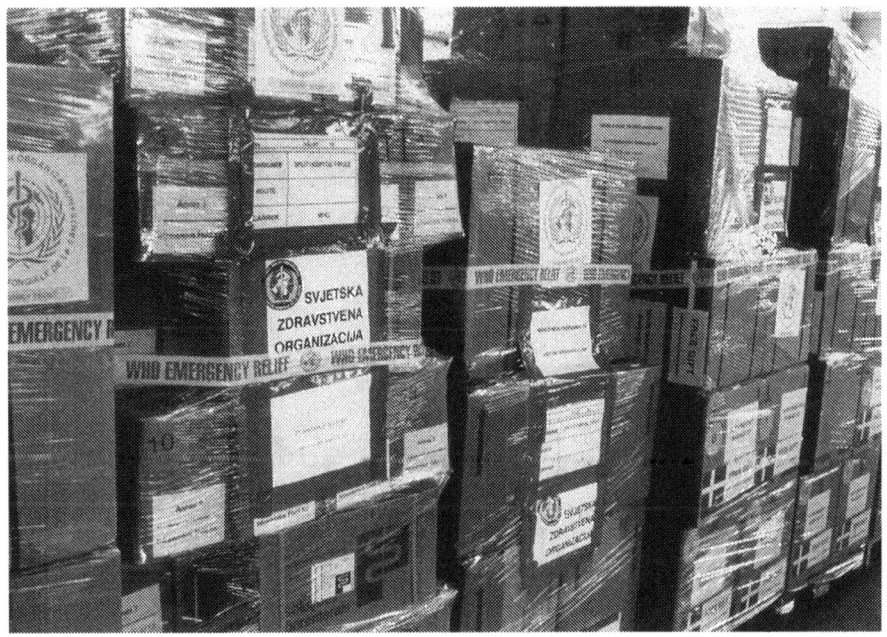

12. W140 Humanitarian relief

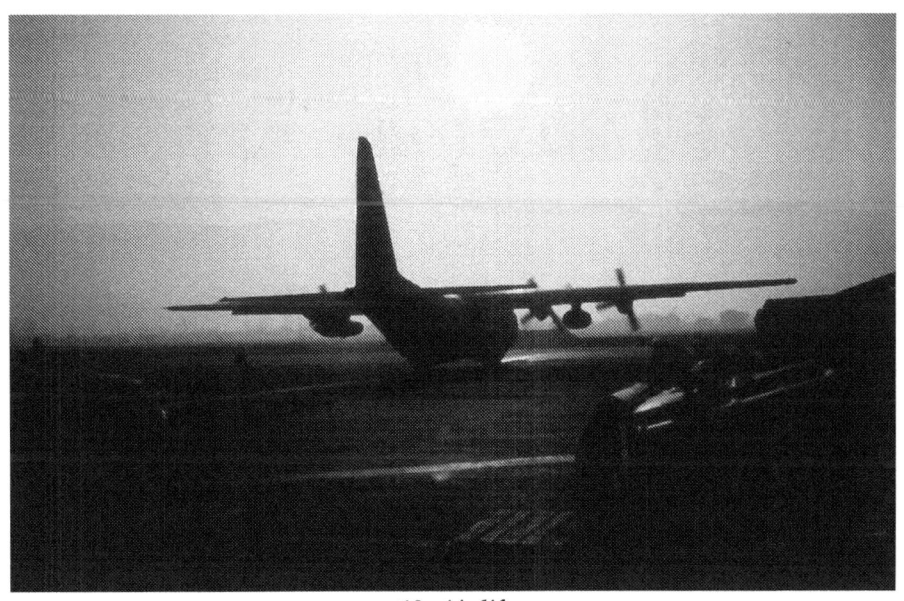

13. Air lift

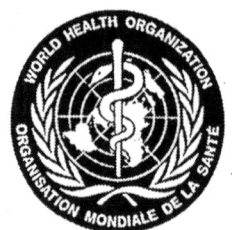

HEALTH MONITOR

*FOR THE WAR AFFECTED
POPULATIONS OF FORMER
YUGOSLAVIA*

Edition No: 4   *18th January 1992*

WINTER PROTECTION

In many parts of the war affected areas of former Yugoslavia buildings are damaged, little fuel is available for heating and cooking, and many people have only meagre supplies of food. It is therefore essential that optimal use is made of the supplies that are available. The advice on winter protection given here is taken from a leaflet recently prepared by WHO entitled "WINTER PROTECTION: HOW TO STAY WARM IN UNHEATED OR POORLY HEATED HOUSES". The advice given is not just that required to ensure survival, but can help all those affected to save energy, and can prevent unnecessary weight loss and reduction of the body's resistance both to cold and to infection.

14. Health monitor – 18th Jan 1992

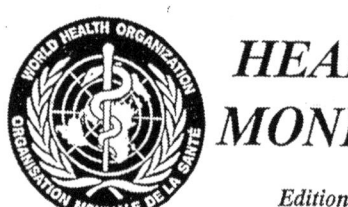

HEALTH MONITOR

*FOR THE WAR AFFECTED
POPULATIONS OF FORMER
YUGOSLAVIA*

Edition No: 2   *20th November 1992*

WATERBORNE INFECTION

In many parts of the war affected areas of former Yugoslavia water purification systems have broken down or have been damaged by the fighting. The risk of contamination of water supplies by pathogenic organisms is therefore high. Large numbers of cases of diarrhoeal illness were reported during the summer and, whilst the number of reports of such infections has declined during the last month, the risk remains high. Typhoid and hepatitis, both of which can be transmitted by water, are causing particular concern at present. Increasing numbers of reports of cases of both these infections have recently been received by WHO.

15. Health monitor – 20th Nov 1992

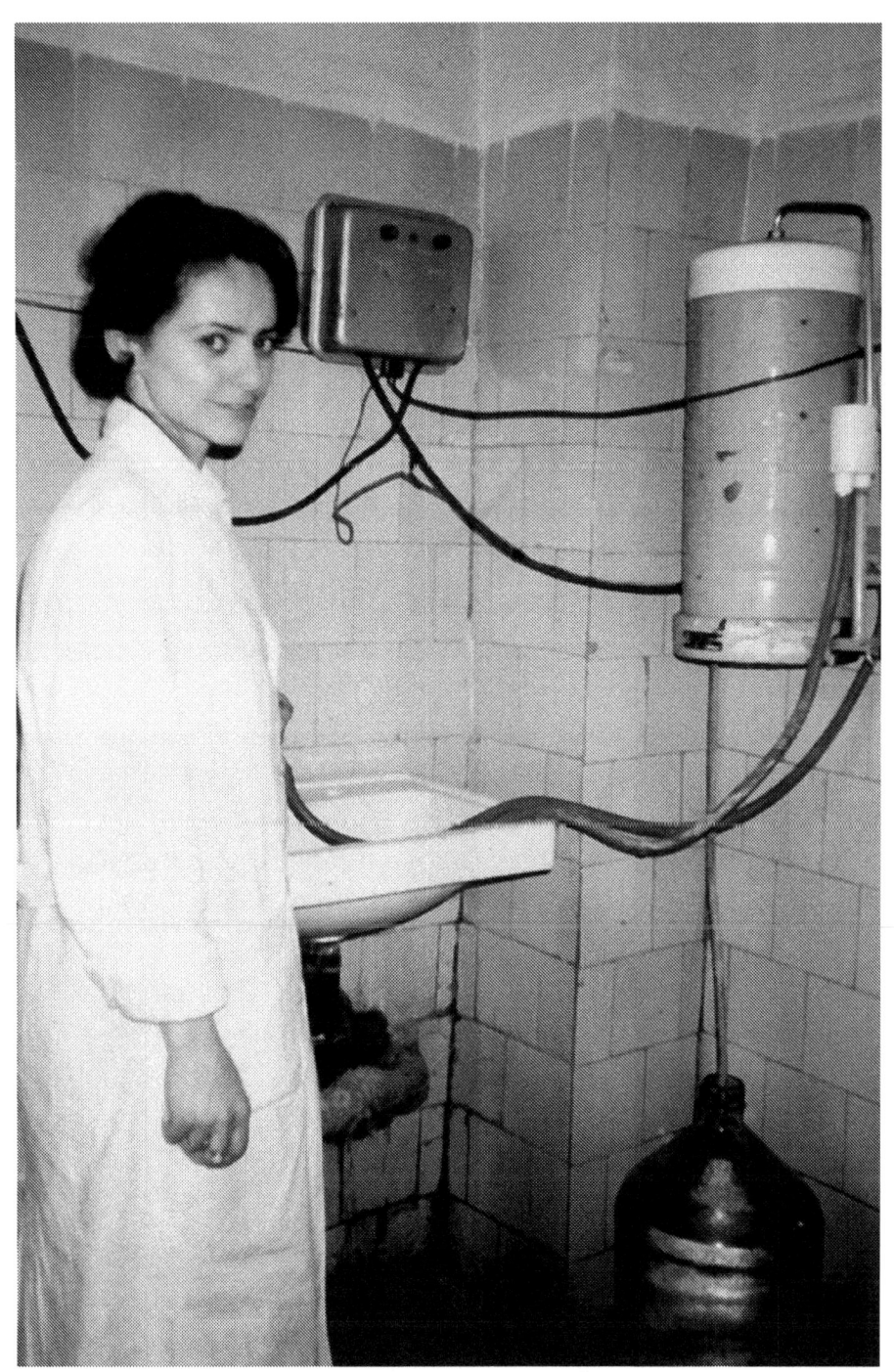

16. Dagestan – no equipment but loving care

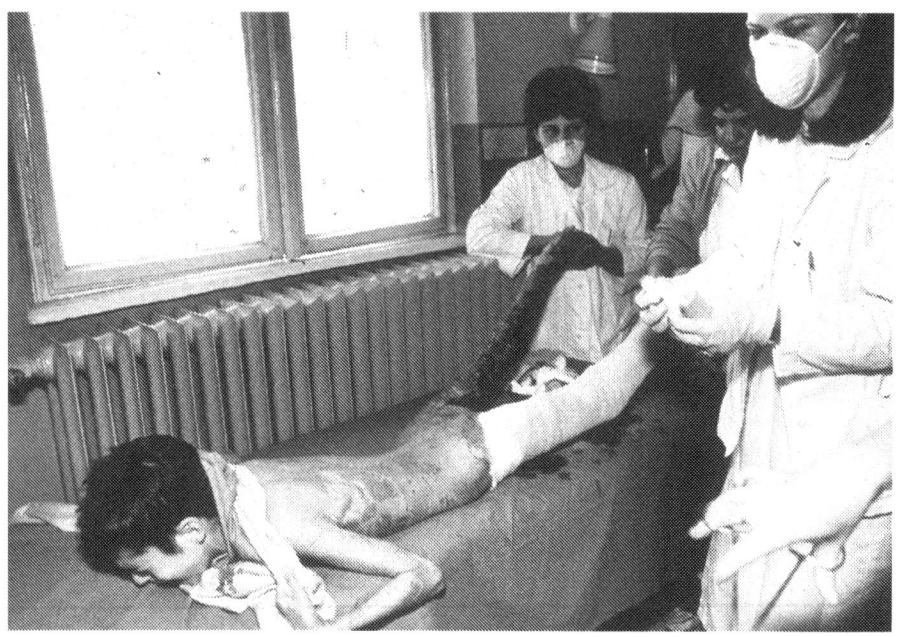

17. Third degree burns, Sarajevo

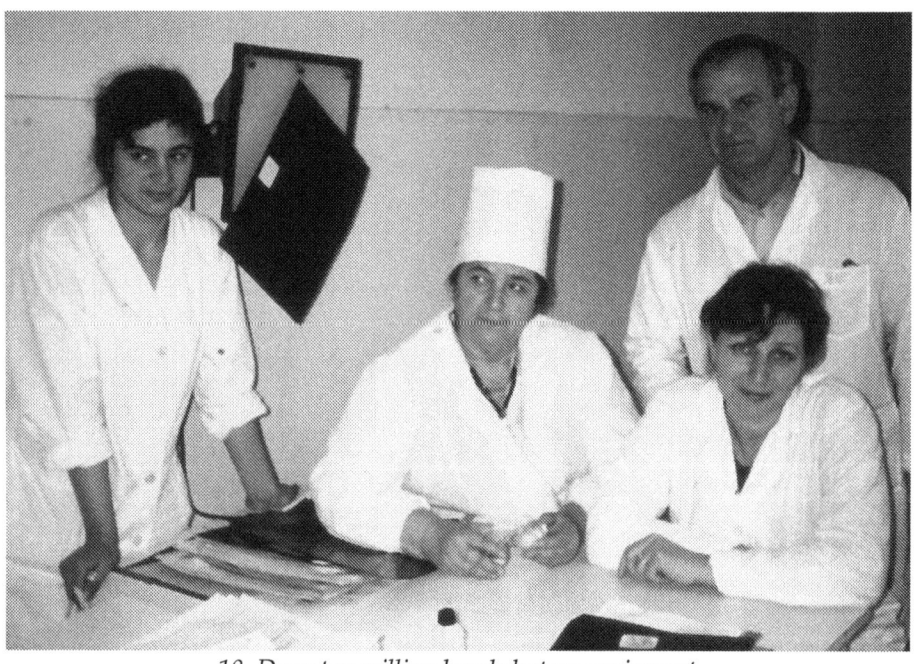

18. Dagestan willing hands but no equipment

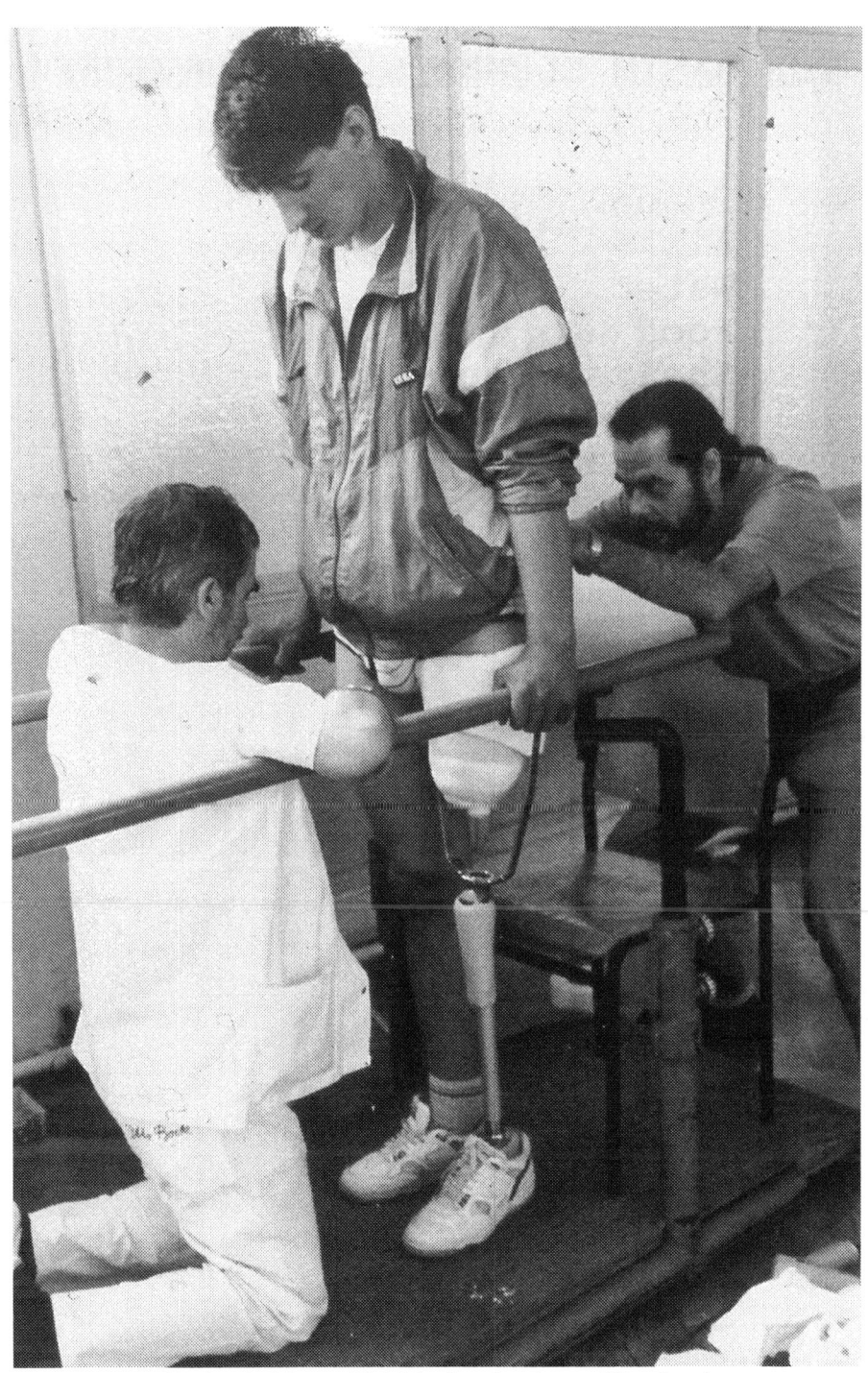

19. *A primitive artificial leg but Sarajevo willing hands*

THE BASIC ELEMENTS FOR SURVIVAL

Peace
Air
Water
Food
Shelter (and fuel)

Medical Supplies

20. The basic elements for survival

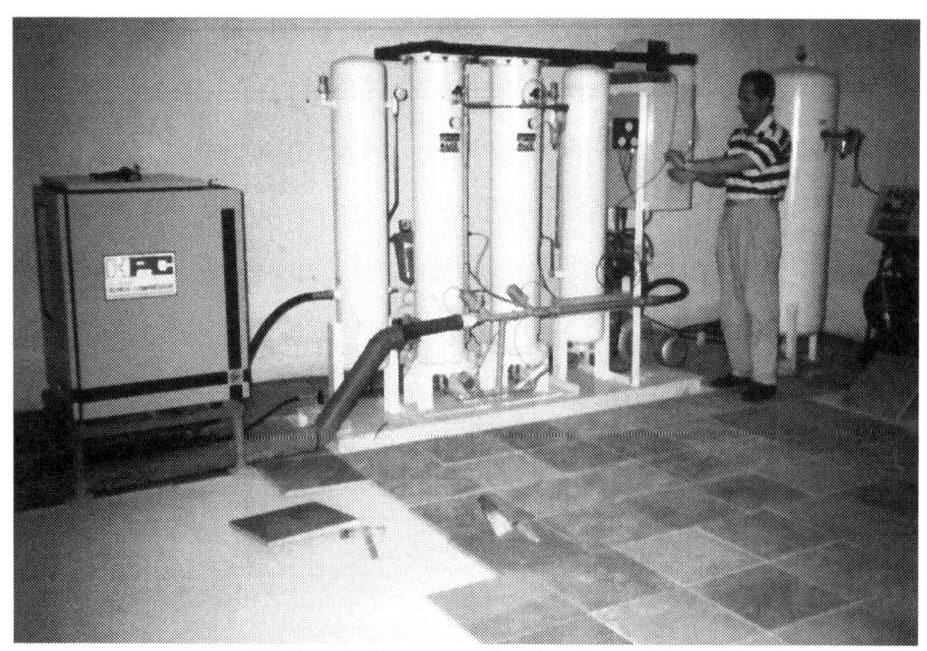

21. Surgical oxygen – Sarajevo basement

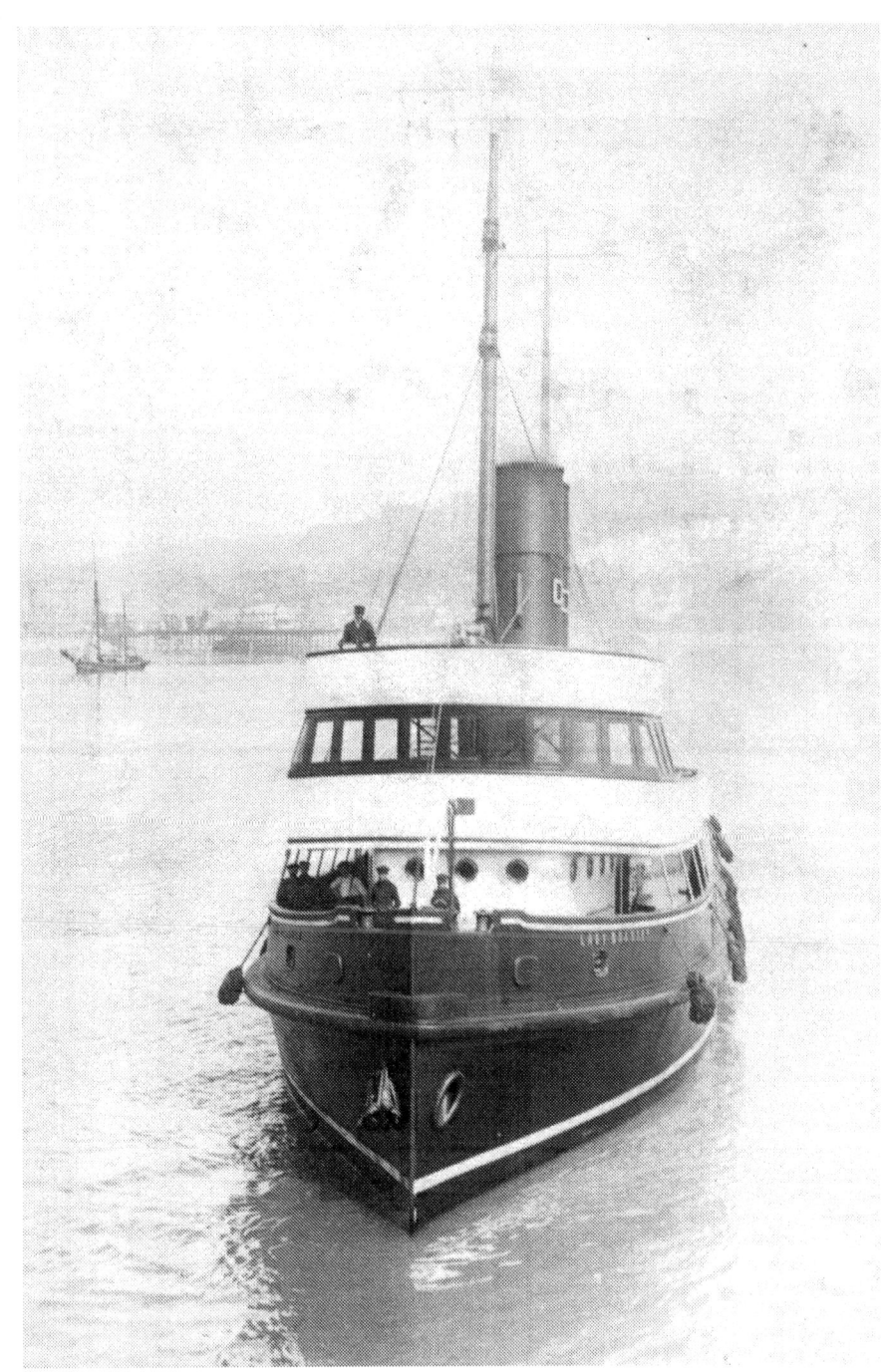

22. My grandfather, Joseph Rennoldson's shipbuilding company built Lady Brassey

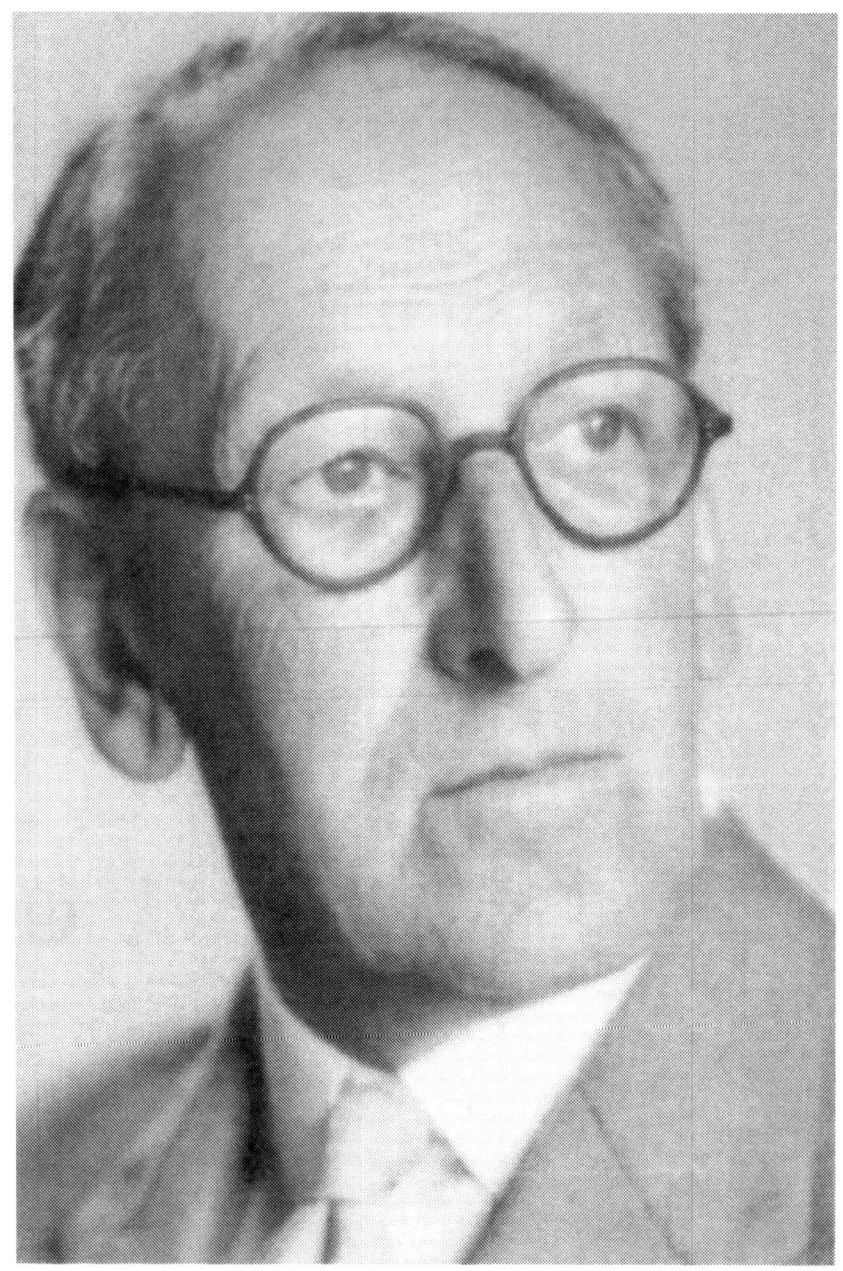

23. Dr Douglas McAlpine – Senior Neurologist, Middlesex Hospital Medical School

CHAPTER 8
A Red Dean for Southampton

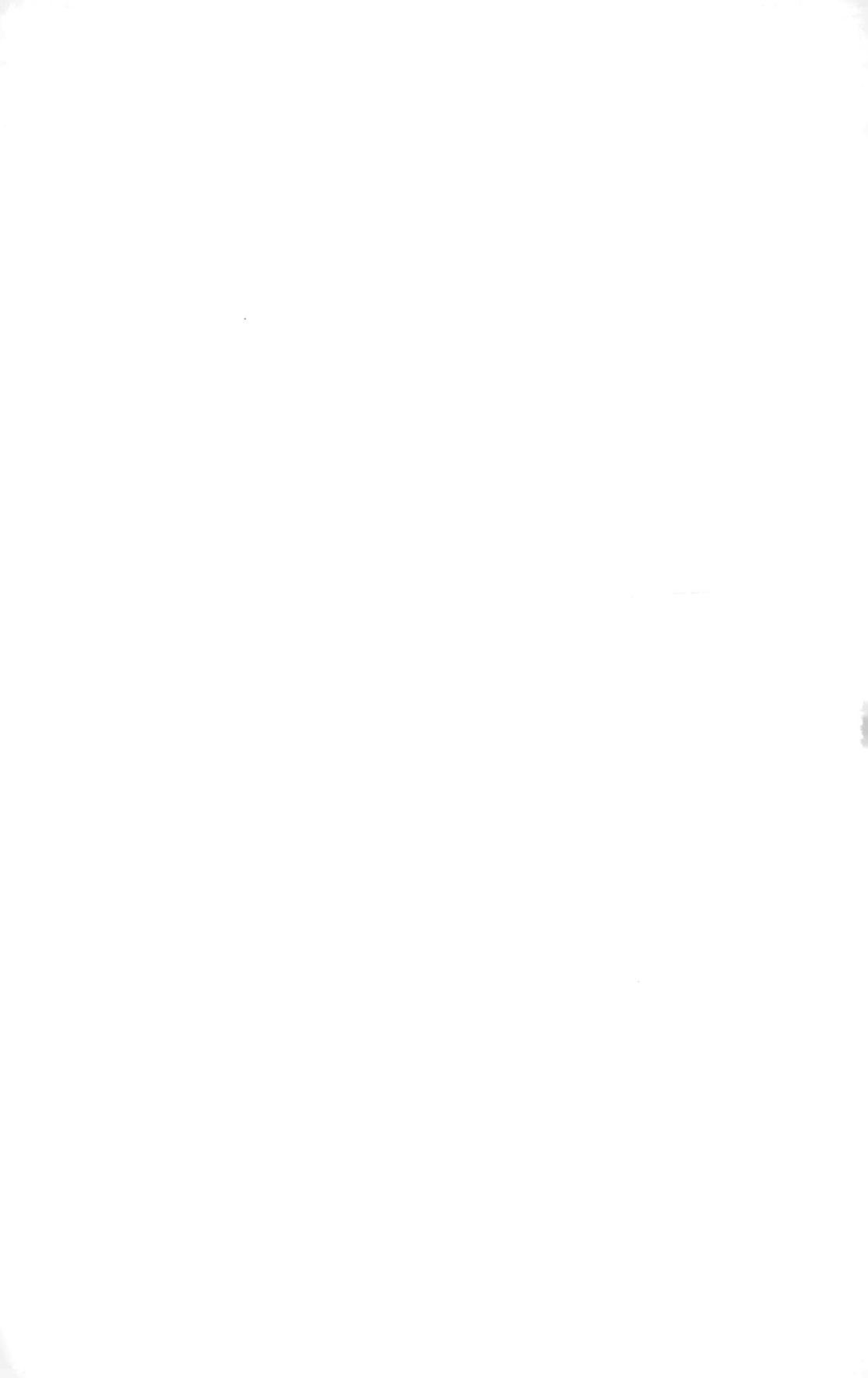

One of the unexplained mysteries of the 20th century is that it was not until 1965 that the existence of a crisis which should have been glaringly obvious for many years dawned upon the government. This was that Britain was training far too few doctors. After all since the earliest days of the NHS in 1948, anyone who needed medical help could not have failed to notice that a large proportion of our doctors were not British but came from the Indian subcontinent or Africa. While some of these were excellent, many suffered from the disadvantage that their home countries simply had not been able to afford the cost of providing modern medical education. Yet, incredible as this now may seem when alarm bells began to ring and the Willink Committee was asked to look at the situation, not only did it come to the wrong conclusion that far from there being too few medical students, there were too many and their numbers should therefore be reduced, but the Government accepted their report and acted upon it.

Fortunately eight years later when the Todd Commission on Medical Education set about its work a wiser view prevailed. This was that the medical manpower question was not only a matter of numbers but also of principle. Todd regarded it as unacceptable that a substantial proportion of the National Health Service's medical staff should have graduated abroad. This time the reversal of opinion led to urgent corrective action. All existing medical schools within the UK were required forthwith to take more students and immediate instructions were given to set up three new schools, respectively at Southampton, Nottingham and Leicester.

It was therefore not surprising that when I arrived in Southampton in 1968 as Dean of the first new Medical School to be established in the United Kingdom for more than half a century, I found mixed with a good deal of excitement a sense of crisis. Nor was it surprising that from that day in 1971 when we managed to provide makeshift facilities and a welcome for our first class of students, we were under intense pressure to expand. Yet thanks to the recruitment of an inspired team of colleagues, and improvisation on a grand scale we were nevertheless able to not only reach our target class size of 130 students by 1976, but also to achieve a formidable series of educational innovations which for twenty-five years have stood the test of time.

But as the old saying points out, it is not possible to make an omelette without breaking eggs and a new medical school, with its colossal scale of need both in terms of buildings and finance in the local hospitals and community as well as within the University, is a very big omelette indeed. That we met with reservations, jealousies and occasionally hostility to begin with was only to be expected. However, most of these subsided when two key issues were clarified. The first was that the additional costs were to be met but not at the expense of the University's existing work but by special funding, and the second that the new academic clinical staff were to practice as equals alongside the various pre-existing NHS consultants in surgery, obstetrics, medicine, etc., not in charge of them.

But in spite of everything, there were occasional misunderstandings. I learned of one of these quite by chance when I attended my first meeting of the Senate a few days after my appointment as Dean. As I was a little late, I was glad to find a seat close to the door, thus saving me the embarrassment of disturbing the discussion. But only a few seconds had passed before I became aware of the reason for the empty seat. My neighbour who was sitting behind a place name marked

'Professor of Philosophy', was busy excavating the evil smelling contents of a particularly foul pipe. He turned to scowl at me.

"And, who may I ask, might you be?" came a stage whisper in a broad Scots accent.

And when I confessed the awful truth:

"Verra bad thing! Verra Bad thing indeed! In Glasgow the Medical School took all our money, and disturbed the whole city with its drunken students! To get away from all that was the only reason I came south!"

His was evidently a deeply felt but fortunately unrepresentative point of view.

But in any case, a medical school needs goodwill and cooperation far beyond the limits of the University. For the clinical part of the course it requires the help of the whole community, patients and doctors alike, and as Southampton is a relatively small city it was necessary for this cooperation to extend beyond it to the whole of Wessex.

Looking back and bearing in mind that the local medical profession had never expected to have a major role in clinical teaching and a few of them had actually chosen to move to Southampton from London to avoid it, the amount of support and enthusiasm we received was remarkable. Admittedly there were a few grumbles particularly at Portsmouth, a larger city than Southampton and a Royal Borough. But this was simply because its doctors had hoped the medical school would be centred there not beside the Solent. In any case these concerns evaporated when Portsmouth's acclaimed centre for the treatment of kidney diseases was given the lead teaching role in that subject in the new school.

Following my arrival in a temporary office in a semi-detached house in University Road, news soon got round that the Todd Report's criticisms had been accepted and that revolutionary new ideas were stirring in Southampton's embryo medical school. It is a tragedy that of the brilliant team who conceived its policies and nurtured its early growth only one, Jack Howell, Professor of Medicine, apart from myself has survived. Only he and I have the satisfaction of knowing how strong the foundations we laid thirty years ago have proved to be. The other pioneers James Frazer the surgeon, David Bulmer the anatomist, David Miller the obstetrician, and Ralph Wright the physician are all now dead.

We asked a great deal of these young men and women, perhaps too much. Not only had they to establish their personal clinical skills as at least the standard of the local specialists – in surgery, psychiatry, obstetrics, etc – but they had to undertake research, be inspiring teachers, help in the creation of a radical new approach to medical education, be diplomatic, and above all - to sustain year on year the creative energy to innovate.

The members of our team, who had been drawn from all parts of the United Kingdom, naturally shared the experience of having themselves been taught as medical students and having taught others. But something else had brought us together. This was profound dissatisfaction with many aspects of the education we ourselves had received and a determination to find a better way. The philosophy we shared was this: to welcome our new students as partners who, with representation on the Faculty Board, would share in the development of the course; to foster their enthusiasm; to help them develop and exploit their own intelligence; and above all, to avoid stuffing them with facts.

While in the early years we had to improvise in hospitals with few facilities for teaching, as pioneers we had a privilege which far outweighed this. As there were no existing staff in a position to form a conservative clique which resisted change, within the broad limits laid down by law through the General Medical Council, we could in effect start from scratch. We took this as a golden opportunity to innovate. As if to declare war on the past and to herald a fresh start we set out two overarching principles: students should start to have meaningful contact with patients immediately in the first year of the course; and at no point should formal teaching by lectures and other classes occupy more than half of the working week. In this way we hoped to capitalise on the enthusiasm which almost all of these gifted young people have on arrival at medical school, sustain it and release a large part of their energies for private studies.

But by far the boldest innovation occurred in the fourth year of the curriculum. In this we incorporated as part of the normal course for all students an opportunity which elsewhere had only been offered to a few at the top of the class who were prepared to spend an additional 'intercalated' year in the university. In contrast the Southampton approach required each and every student to devote six months of their fourth year to planning and carrying out an original investigation under supervision; to write it up and to present it for critical discussion to the whole class of fellow students at the end of the year.

Even in the early years when on 'The Fourth Year Day' in June, sixty or seventy students each presented the results of their personal projects in a series of ten-minute communications, I found it an extraordinary and inspiring experience. But now that the class consists of two hundred students, it has become not only an intellectual tour de force but a logistic miracle.

Our object is that in the 'fourth year' students should not only discover that most medical knowledge is based on science but far more important that it is often uncertain and indeed hypothetical and in clinical practice at all times requires critical evaluation. We felt that the sheer volume of the facts which medical students have to absorb leads to these often being presented as oversimplified half-truths. In other words, the uncertainty surrounding much accepted knowledge remains concealed.

A project undertaken by a fourth year student may consist of a piece of original research, a review, or a survey relating to any part of the curriculum. In practice the scope has proved to be enormous. Although, as might be expected, standards have varied, some have achieved publication, others more modestly finding a place in the medical school library. But whatever the standard, the object is achieved if the student concludes it with a more realistic view of the limitations of received knowledge, a sharpened critical faculty when in future he makes choices on behalf of his patients and some skill and confidence when speaking in public. Concealed within the genesis of the Southampton 'fourth year' was also, I like to think, a germ of my own seminal experience many years previously at Oxford. This was when my tutor, Percy O'Brien, having first told me not to worry about attending all the lectures, set me my first essay:

"You'll find the library in Parks' Road – here are a few references,"

and, concluded with the words which fifty years later still ring in my ears,

"the ball's in your court now!"

In the early years the 'Fourth Year Day' culminated in a nautical celebration known as the 'River Boat Shuffle'. After all, students who had borne several months of increasing pressure in preparing their first piece of original research, and had then plucked up the courage to deliver the results to a large audience felt the need of a party. It became a custom that the Medical School hired a Solent ferry boat complete with bar, restaurant, and dance floor and all of us, students and staff alike, set out on a trip to the Isle of Wight and back with a break on the Island for refreshments. To begin with, all went well at these maritime parties, but as the years went by and the student numbers increased what had started as a more or less intimate affair became more and more uproarious.

In 1977 with about 100 students ready to 'let off steam' and half as many staff on board, the 'shuffle' finally came to grief. As the boat neared the Isle of Wight, various people dived overboard, swam ashore and invaded the local pubs. The climax came when the boat was about to leave on the return trip. Some of the students succeeded in purloining[17] a barrel of beer from one of the pubs. The police were called and I found myself in the Island's only police station bailing them out. We all got home safely but that was the end of the 'River Boat Shuffle.' Looking back, it was providential that no one was drowned.

---

[17] This theft was possible because the Isle of Wight at that time was the only place in the English speaking world where pubs had no 'bar' separating the customers from the liquor including beer barrels and the publican.

A pause for reflection

The year 1976 was for me in many ways a climax in which I felt a glow of attainment but at the same time a sense of exhaustion. The first small class of students, although they sometimes complained of having been experimented on like guinea pigs, had been partners in an extraordinary adventure in which they had played a crucial and constructive role. All passed their finals at the first attempt. In the second year the school reached its target quota of 130 new entrants. Just before I stepped down as Dean and handed over to Jack Howell, we had a visit from Sir George Pickering, Regius Professor at Oxford. George was in those days the doyen of academic medicine. He chose to visit us while touring medical schools in preparation for a book. Here are two excerpts of his Report:

"The boldest and in many ways the most successful new curriculum is that of the University of Southampton."

"I would like to hazard the opinion that this venture of Southampton's is the most important experiment in medical education in my lifetime. It should provide the young graduate with the discipline and habits of mind of the scholar, and thus fit him for the opportunity of self education which he will enjoy ... for the rest of his life."

In the twenty-five years since George Pickerings' Report, the Medical School at Southampton has continued to grow and thrive. Today with an entry quota of 200 students a year its 3,000 graduates are practising medicine in all parts of the English-speaking world.

Research has also flourished. In at least three widely different fields – the relationship of the growth of the foetus in vitro to the occurrence of coronary heart disease in later life; of asthma to the inflammation of the airways and in the study of Burkitt's lymphoma in Uganda – it has gained international distinction. This has been recognised in a Millennial Award for clinical research from the Wellcome Foundation.

The new medical school at Brighton has been invited by the General Medical Council to base its curriculum on Southampton's Medical School as a model, making whatever modifications they please. In a national survey by medical students of their schools, Southampton has come top. The school continues to make provision for mature and graduate students and 50 of the 240 places are set aside for these to take a special accelerated course. If there is a disadvantage associated with all these successes, it is that the academic requirement for entry has had to be increased to 2 A' and a B' at A Level.

But the brilliance of Southampton's Medical School was no 'flash in the pan'. At the turn of the 20th century almost thirty years after the entry of the first class of medical students, further independent reviews took place. In both teaching and research Southampton received the highest possible grade.

The Red Dean

And how did I achieve my nickname? Not I think because of a mistaken view that I was a member of the Communist Party nor I suspect because of the unorthodox curriculum. I think the nickname almost certainly stemmed from our chosen method of selecting students from the many applicants. We were, I believe, the first medical school not to interview but to rely exclusively on a report from the school and examination results. We did this because we could find no objective evidence that interviewing seventeen year olds provided a reliable guide to their suitability for a medical career. We also suspected that at interviews unconscious bias might lead us to favour unfairly young men and women with like backgrounds, manners, and deportment to ourselves.

On an occasion when I tried to explain our approach at a meeting with the wives of members of the Wessex branch of the BMA – adding with a singular lack of tact that there would be no special favours for those with a medical parent. I was received not only with disbelief but in stony silence. Perhaps ironically the BMA ladies had not grasped another equally radical aspect of our admissions policy which might have pleased them. Ours was to be one of the first schools in the UK to reject the prevalent policy of providing only a small quota of places for female students and to admit women on equal terms to men.

But there may have been another reason for my 'Red Dean' nickname. This was my enthusiasm at that time for the idea that medical education should be added to the courses provided by the Open University, an institution which had recently been created to enable part time 'mature' students to work for University degrees from their homes while continuing meantime, to earn their living. Two aspects of my experience as Dean at Southampton had led me to this view.

The first and foremost was my meeting with large numbers of able mature men and women from all strata of society for all of whom we could not find places, whose burning desire almost to the point of obsession was to become a doctor but who for various reasons had not gained a place in the orthodox way at the end of their secondary education. Secondly, I had become convinced that the range of skills and aptitudes required in modern medicine was too diverse to be met by what almost amounted to a clone of young men and women however brilliant, selected at the age of seventeen principally for their ability in the sciences and mathematics. This persuaded me that there was a need for diversification of entry to the medical profession to help

with the national imbalance of medical manpower in relation to the number and nature of the jobs within it. While training for acute surgery, medicine and obstetrics was oversubscribed, other important areas had far too few trainees.

Notable among the so-called 'Cinderella' specialities at that time were the care of the aged, certain branches of psychiatry and of pathology and the care of people with sexually transmitted disease. There were also marked geographical differences, with severe shortages of the less popular specialities in the North and West while the wealthy and comfortable South and West were oversubscribed.

To have chosen this of all topics as the subject of a high profile visiting lecture at of all places the ultra conservative city of Bath showed an astonishing lack of 'savoir faire' and tact on my part – which even thirty year later makes me blush. Nevertheless although startled and cool, they were polite. Today, the Open University tell me it still adheres to its policy not to provide courses to prepare students for a medical career. I find this disappointing.

A new adventure

Having handed over the post of Dean to Jack Howell, and spent a sabbatical year at McMaster University in Ontario, I returned to Southampton in 1978 much refreshed. What would happen next? After all, I had only just turned fifty. Would I be invited to become Vice-Chancellor somewhere or would there be an opportunity outside academic life, for example, in the civil service or the pharmaceutical industry? Once again my career was to take an unexpected turn following the arrival of a letter marked 'Strictly Private and Confidential.'

On that occasion the letter proved to be from no lesser a personage than Sir James Gowans, who at that time was Secretary to the Medical Research Council, arguably the most distinguished research organisation in the world. It contained an invitation set in astonishing terms. Subject only to my submitting detailed proposals, I was invited to set up a new Research Unit in Environmental Epidemiology "on any subject you care to choose and in association with any University within the United Kingdom you consider appropriate."[18] As I look back after all these years it is crystal clear that this extraordinary compliment was more a tribute to my flair for attracting talented people and for organisation than recognition of my modest research in occupational cancer. I accepted it with enthusiasm.

The decision about the location of the Unit was easy to make. It was obvious it should be in Southampton. I already had an outstanding team there and I knew for a fact that the presence of the Medical Research Council there was welcome both to the University and the City. As for the focus of our work, it seemed commonsense to base it on the two lines of research on which my friend David Barker and I were already working.

These were, in David's case, the extraordinary geographical pattern of diseases such as coronary heart disease and diabetes; and as far as I was concerned, what happened to the health of various industrial workers who had been exposed to chemicals which may cause cancer and to various types of dust.

---

[18] The invitation was based on a decision made by the MRC at the meeting of Council in November 1978.

For me, these seemingly very different lines of inquiry were linked. Thus I recalled that when I was working at Oxford it had been the discovery of an unexpected cluster of cases of nasal cancer in Northamptonshire that provided me with the first hint that this disease was not found exclusively among furniture workers. Sure enough when we looked into it further we found that these malignant tumours also occurred in the boot and shoe industry but limited to men whose job was to use high speed grinding machines to shape the special leather, hardened by tanning, which is used for soles and heels.

Likewise an important part of the case against the use of blue asbestos (crocidolite) which led to its prohibition was also based on geography. Thus the geographical distribution of mesothelioma – the fatal cancer of the lining of the chest and abdomen – corresponded almost exactly with the location of the pre-war naval shipyards in which, because of its superior fire-resisting qualities, it was preferred as compared to the less dangerous but also less effective white asbestos – chrysotile.

But the asbestos story has another fascinating twist which shows how in epidemiology as in other fields exceptions can help prove a rule. In the MRC unit as we mapped the pattern of deaths from mesothelioma in England in the 1970's, we found clear evidence of an epidemic still occurring in a small Lancashire town many miles from any shipyard. A factory situated there, but long since closed, had manufactured gas masks for the Armed Forces during World War Two. These had contained crocidolite acknowledged to be the most effective filter for protection against poison gas in war.

What about the civilian gas masks which had been manufactured on a much greater scale – one of which had been issued to me as a schoolboy? I traced their manufacture to another town in Lancashire where no cases of mesothelioma had been reported. It turned out that in these masks, the less effective but cheaper (and much safer) white asbestos, chrysotile had been used.

The history of asbestos in the UK has an ironic, indeed a tragic postscript. By the time Britain went to war with Argentina over the Falklands war in 1982, asbestos of all kinds had been banned for use on health grounds as a protection against fire in the Royal Navy. Alas, when HMS Sheffield was struck by an Argentine missile she burned fiercely with many casualties.

Other hazards at work

After I left the MRC Environmental Epidemiology Unit in 1983, to become Chief Medical Officer, the research there on occupational health hazards was continued by Martin Gardner and David Coggon. For some time the main focus, as when I was Director, was on known and suspected occupational causes of cancer. Studies were conducted on workers exposed to various substances including formaldehyde, man-made mineral fibres, phenoxyl acid herbicides, styrene, ethylene oxide and mineral acid mists. In many cases, the data obtained were later collated with information from similar studies, in other countries in collaborative investigations coordinated by the International Agency for Research on Cancer, allowing stronger conclusions to be drawn. As most of these studies showed little evidence of a cancer hazard, even in workers who had been heavily exposed to the chemical of concern, they gave valuable reassurance that use of important new technologies could safely continue.

Subsequently, attention turned also to health effects other than cancer which industrial exposure might produce. One of these was the discovery of a previously unrecognised hazard of infectious pneumonia from occupational exposure to metal fume. In the early 1990s, the Unit was contracted to carry out a new national analysis of occupational mortality for the Health and Safety Executive and the Office of Population Censuses and Surveys. Such analyses are performed approximately every 10 years, and findings from earlier periods had suggested unusually high death rates from pneumonia in welders. The new investigation not only confirmed this, but also showed that the high risks extended to other occupations involving exposure to metal fume, for example in foundries; but it was principally for lobar pneumonia; and that it was confined to deaths occurring before the normal retirement age of 65 years. This pointed strongly to a short-term, reversible increase in susceptibility to pneumonic infection, an idea that was supported by a later study focussed on men admitted to hospital with pneumonia. Research on this problem is now directed towards understanding the biological processes that underlie the hazard.

Since 1985, the Unit has also become a major centre for epidemiological research on occupational causes of musculoskeletal disease. A series of studies demonstrated a marked increase in the risk of hip osteoarthritis among farmers, which appeared to be due to frequent lifting and carrying. Similar findings emerged from parallel studies in other countries, and this culminated in a recent recommendation from the Industrial Injuries Advisory Council that hip osteoarthritis in farmers should be classed as an occupational disease attracting compensation. Other studies in the unit have pointed to risks of knee osteoarthritis and knee cartilage injury from long occupational kneeling; and major progress has been made in trying to disentangle the complex interplay of physical, psychological and social influences that contribute to the enormous burden of disability and sickness absence currently from back pain.

Over the past 30 years, the capacity for occupational health research in British universities has declined significantly, and because of this, the MRC's investment in this area in Southampton has increased in importance.

David Barker and 'The Barker Hypothesis'

When in 1968 I arrived in Southampton to set up the Medical School, I insisted that I should have facilities to enable me to continue my clinical work as a consultant physician. Some beds were found for me at the Royal South Hants Hospital and I was soon taking my turn on the rota of physicians who were responsible for the care of emergency admissions from the city and the surrounding area. Not only did I enjoy the diversion clinical work gave me from planning and administration but the clinical link was important for another reason. It helped the new School gain credibility with the local doctors who, as they were beginning to realise, would soon be taking a major rôle in teaching our students.

For a while this arrangement worked well. But following the arrival of the first class of students in 1971, it rapidly became unsustainable. I urgently needed to find a partner who would not only share my clinical responsibilities but would also strengthen the research team in the newly founded department of epidemiology.

David Barker, who in 1972 joined me as a physician at the Royal South Hants Hospital, has turned out to be much more than a sound clinician. As a research scientist, the originality of his ideas on human growth and development has put him in the same class as the great Victorian inventors Snow and Lind whose work led to the purification of drinking water and the discovery of vitamins. Like theirs in our day David Barker's work has 'broken the mould' of scientific thought for some of the most prevalent diseases of our time. David has shown that coronary heart disease, high blood pressure and diabetes while in part due to lifestyle in adult life actually have their roots in disturbances in the growth of the foetus in the womb and in early infancy.

But as these disturbances also influence the development of the brain and the skeleton, David Barker's work has even wider implications. Thus retarded infant growth may slow the development of the brain and lead to impairment of cognitive function, and in turn to lower occupational status and income. Babies who are small at birth also have lighter bones and a greater tendency to suffer fractures in later life.

These findings have social and educational implications extending far beyond the craft of clinical medicine. It is now clearer than ever thanks to Barker's recent discoveries that young women, the mothers of the future, occupy a role crucial not only to the health of their own children but to the nation's future health. Schools and colleges must help by adapting and strengthening the curriculum, the key being that all young women should have a clear view of their responsibilities and how to meet them by providing not only themselves but their children born and unborn with a healthy diet. They should eat more fruit and vegetables, rice and pasta, fish and wholemeal bread, and less crisps, sweets, cakes and biscuits, red and processed meat, chips and sugar.

An interesting aspect of David Barker's work has been its dependence not on experiments in a laboratory but on the careful labours of past generations of midwives and health visitors. Their painstaking efforts in measuring and recording data about generations of babies in the early years of the twentieth century, have almost a hundred years later, laid the foundations of a veritable revolution in our understanding of the origins of good health. The debate which has emerged is now global in scale. A World Congress on the Foetal Origins of Disease was held in India in 2001. A second such congress took place in 2003.

In 1983, too close for the comfort of my conscience to the opening date of the magnificent building which had just been provided by the MRC for the Southampton Unit, I was presented once again with an opportunity which was impossible to refuse. This time it came about not by means of a letter marked 'Private and Confidential', but with a smile and a handshake across the Whitehall desk of the Secretary to the Cabinet, Sir Robert Armstrong. I had been appointed Chief Medical Officer of England.

CHAPTER 9
Whitehall as I found it

When one foggy morning in October 1983 I arrived at the Department of Health and Social Security (DHSS) to start work as Chief Medical Officer, I discovered that I was the first person recruited from outside the Civil Service to occupy the post since the legendary Wilson Jamieson had steered Britain through the crisis of the Second World War. As, like him, I was an academic I had only the vaguest notion how a great Department of State in Whitehall worked. I felt uncertain of myself and almost as nervous as I had been when as a child I first went off to boarding school. I had no previous experience of the Civil Service except through my father who had been Chief Medical Adviser to the Ministry of Pensions in Northern Ireland. His experience had shown me that working as a medical civil servant was interesting, secure in terms of salary and pension, and prestigious

Fortunately for me, an old friend was there to bid me welcome. My predecessor who was just stepping down was none other than Henry Yellowlees with whom many years previously I had worked closely as Resident Medical Officer at the Middlesex Hospital. As Henry picked up his briefcase and donned his hat and coat, his words of counsel lost nothing from the fact that he was the son of a well-known psychiatrist.

"You'll enjoy this job, Donald, there's never a dull moment! But," he went on, "a word in your ear! Treat the Ministers exactly as you would patients suffering from stress – that's basically what they are! As for the officials, the system works like clockwork. If you listen to them they'll keep you from falling into any of Whitehall's 'elephant traps'."

I took his advice.

Before he left Henry had one more point to make as he began to remove what I thought was a framed modernist picture from the wall.

"You're going, inevitably to lose control of your life, I'm afraid! Look at this! It isn't a picture, its four tickets for Aida at Covent Garden last year, booked ages in advance to celebrate my birthday. We never got there! Instead, at the last minute and in my black tie, I spent the evening counselling a Minister who was in a panic about a speech in the Commons the next day."

I came in at the top of an hierarchical system of which my predecessor had, as was customary, worked his way up from the bottom rung. There was method and indeed considerable strength in this remarkable system. It ensured that the CMO when he gave advice to Ministers or the public could do so with a degree of authority far beyond his personal expertise. Fortunately I had an extensive range of expert advisers who together covered every aspect of public health and clinical practice. This ensured that when a Question was asked in the House of Commons about a topical problem whether for example salmonella in eggs or the excessive waiting list for surgical operations in Hull, I could call upon someone to brief me at short notice on any issue which might be raised in Parliament or the media.

My awesome range of responsibility was exemplified by my experience in the first few weeks which included advising whether the new nuclear reactor at Sellafield was responsible for a local cluster of cases of leukaemia, whether it was safe to put chlorine in drinking water, and whether it was appropriate to withdraw Welfare Milk which had been supplied free as a dietary supplement to poor children since before the war. At the same time, the need for doctors in Whitehall was being questioned by the Prime Minister as part of her strategy to downsize government.

But there were aspects of the job which needed time for adjustment, and which recalled my brief period in the Armed Forces. Almost before I had sat down at my desk for the first time, I was asked to read and sign the 'Official Secrets Act'. My relaxed persona as an academic disappeared even further into the distance when I found out that I had now become a 'Grade 1(a) Civil Servant' with some sixty or more doctors in Grades 2,3,4,5, etc., 'in my command'. I also discovered that working alongside these doctors was a parallel administrative hierarchy of career civil servants also Graded 2,3,4,5,etc. who were answerable to Sir Kenneth Stowe, the Permanent Secretary. He, in the most helpful way possible as it turned out, was also in charge of me! This chapter is written with due regard to that confidentiality.

Another aspect of the work was more difficult for a newcomer to understand. This was an extraordinary degree of secrecy over what appeared to be relatively mundane matters together with paranoia about unauthorised 'leaks'. After all, the Department did not deal with defence or foreign policy but with health and social services. An issue which came up within a few weeks of my arrival was a case in point. There was a need for the public purse to make savings, and free 'welfare' milk for school children cost approximately the amount required. Now, fifty years after milk tokens had been introduced to help the hungry, rickety children of the thirties, was it safe to give it up? My immediate reaction was to turn to my expert advisor at Great Ormond Street for advice.

"Sorry, you can't do that!" I was horrified to hear, "Far too risky!" That way the matter might leak to the Press before Ministers have made up their mind."

So having been thrown in at the deep end, I had the choice to sink or swim. Fortunately, my largely untutored recommendation turned out to be correct. It was that with the improvements in diet during and since the war and the virtual disappearance of rickets, welfare milk could now safely be withdrawn.

But the technical aspects of health were only part of the story. As I settled in, another impression began to emerge. This was of a Department covering such an enormous scale of work – which at that time included not only the National Health Service and the social services but the social security system as well - that it was, I sensed, seriously overworked, and with the best will in the world was beginning to creak under the strain. On the shoulders of the Permanent Secretary Sir Kenneth Stowe fell the responsibility not only of running the Department but of accounting to Parliament for the whole of the gigantic expenditure, amounting in those days to more than £50 billion per annum. Although I could not myself have managed the finances of a winkle stall, I insisted in giving him at least my moral support. Thus I went along with him to attend regular inquisitions about the finances of the National Health Service which he suffered at the hands of the Public Accounts Committee of the House of Commons.

But at a time when parliamentary sessions often continued throughout the night, it was not we Civil Servants, but Ministers and in particular the Secretary of State on whom the heaviest burden fell. Although I saw four Secretaries of State come and go, it was Norman

Fowler with whom I worked for several years who I got to know best. Ours was a productive partnership which included not only the largely successful policies for the control of HIV/AIDS, legionellosis and salmonellosis but the revival of public health. Norman's success was based on a rare capacity to choose the right priorities together with the self-discipline to pursue them single-mindedly to a conclusion. Here is an example how his careful attention to detail was often decisive. Having read my paper proposing an Inquiry 'into the public health function' he sent for me. As we sat down together he smiled and took out his pen.

"Not an inquiry into the public health function, Donald," he said, "let's be much more upbeat! 'An Inquiry into the future development of the public health function' is what we need."

And so due to Norman Fowler's apparently trivial alteration in its title, the possibility of a negative outcome went out of the window and the consequence of the inquiry was eventually a renaissance of public health not only within the United Kingdom but by imitation in many other parts of the English-speaking world and which has been sustained to the present day.

The Government's Doctor

During my eight years in Whitehall I worked closely with no fewer than four Secretaries of State – Norman Fowler, Kenneth Clarke, John Moore and William Waldegrave as well as with a host of other Ministers in their teams including the future Prime Minister, John Major. While all the Ministers happened to be Conservatives due to the period, I never thought of them in party terms. For me they were public servants carrying heavy responsibilities, working to an impossible schedule, under almost intolerable strain. At a time when the Department covered not only the NHS but Social Security and Social Services, Senior Ministers in addition to meetings of the Cabinet and its subcommittees and constituency duties, had to attend a House of Commons which in those days kept intolerable hours, including all night sessions.

Although as a civil servant I was totally impartial in political terms, as someone who had recently retired from clinical practice I found myself following my predecessor Henry Yellowlees advice and thinking of Ministers as patients under pressure. Short of actual medical treatment, I tried to give them as much support and encouragement as I could.

Perhaps my greatest compliment came at a relaxed moment from Kenneth Clark.

"Do you know, Donald, we've worked together all these years and I haven't the slightest notion which way you vote?"

For a moment I was quite taken aback. Was he asking a question which was out of bounds?

To tell him would be wrong in principle; not to answer would be rude. Fortunately my Ulster upbringing came to my help.

"At the time of the Irish Question, my grandfather was a strong supporter of Mr Gladstone",

I said with a twinkle in my eye. We both laughed and the moment passed.

The luck of the Irish

Luck perhaps helped by a modicum of good management brought me two successes early in my Whitehall career which helped establish my reputation with Ministers. The problems could not have been more different. One was a serious outbreak of illness in babies, the other a major showdown between the government and the British Medical Association.

Early in the autumn of 1985 news began to arrive in my office in Alexander Fleming House of a number of mysterious cases of gastroenteritis in infants. Tragically some of these had proved fatal. The pattern of the outbreak was unusual because the cases did not occur among newborn babies in poor families but after weaning and right across the social spectrum. Most mysterious of all was that the microbe identified in the sick children, <u>Salmonella ealing</u>, had previously only been found in, of all places - seagulls.

Fortunately, within the Department we had a group of experts – the 'environmental health officers' (EHOs) - whose job it was to don the mantle of Sherlock Holmes as far as food hygiene was concerned. They made urgent visits to the homes of the affected infants and to those of an equal number of well babies born in the same districts over the same period. This led to an interesting discovery. 'Ostermilk', manufactured by 'Farley Foods', seemed to be associated with the illness. The trouble was that the association was not strong enough to be conclusive, and worse no sign of Salmonella ealing could be found in samples of the milk.

Sitting in my office in Alexander Fleming House where by this time almost fifty cases had been reported and new cases were appearing daily, I found myself in a very difficult position. Should I wait for more evidence; or take the plunge and broadcast a warning not to use Farley Infant Food? It did not need a legal genius to realise that if we proved wrong and unnecessarily bankrupted the firm, we would face an unpleasant lawsuit and probably exemplary damages.

After a sleepless night I decided to put the case to Barney Hayhoe, at that time the Minister of Health. Should things go wrong it would be Barney who would formally be accountable to Parliament for the mistake. But I would not escape blame and would almost certainly get the sack. Providence seemed to be smiling on me when it turned out that Barney had studied statistics at university.

Together we poured over the figures again and again. Even with an additional case the next day, the odds in favour of Farley Foods being the culprit did not quite reach formal statistical significance. But if the outbreak was not due to Farley Foods, what else could be the cause? Asking that question cleared our minds. There were no other contenders. The same day I used TV and radio to warn the public the sale of Ostermilk was prohibited, and it was removed from the shops.

Slowly, all too slowly as it seemed to me, the number of reports of illness began to decline. Had we made a terrible mistake I asked myself, as I tossed and turned in bed at night? If the mysterious microbe found in the sick children was not in Ostermilk, where had it come from? Seemingly an age later the mystery was solved. The scrutiny of the Farley Foods factory in Lancashire had almost been completed when Salmonella ealing was found. It was present in seagull droppings in the high level tank which supplied water to the plant.

The 'limited list'

A quite different part of the CMO's job, and one which I was singularly ill-prepared for was to act as the 'go-between', or in pompous diplomatic terms, as the 'interlocutor' when disputes arose between the Government which is paymaster of almost all the doctors in the land and the British Medical Association which acts as their trade union.

Fortunately when it came to the negotiation of salaries it was my administrative friends in the Department who dealt with it. But from time to time other problems arose which, using civil service slang, brought the CMO 'into play'.

In the case in point, the issue was the cost of the NHS at a time when the country was struggling against inflation and mounting external debt. Across government, all Departments were asked to find savings and in the DHSS the target we were set was £100m per annum. But where could such a large sum be found without compromising patient care, that was the question?

At this distance in time, I am not sure whether the notion that the huge bill for medicines might be an area for savings was mine or someone else's. What is certain is that I thought it was a good idea. As someone who had myself practiced as a clinician in the NHS for many years I knew that not all medicines in use had been proved to be effective. Also even with those of proven efficacy there was often a large gap in cost between 'name brand' drugs and their generic equivalent. I was also aware of the unseemly pressure that was sometimes put on doctors to prescribe the more expensive patented variety, for example, 'Valium' or 'Aspro' rather than the cheaper generic product 'diazepam' or 'aspirin'. For many years it had been commonplace for drug companies to sponsor lectures and seminars in hospitals and postgraduate centres: the cold buffet being provided by the company in return for an arrangement to display its wares. The 'detail man' as the salesman of the particular drug company was called, had become a familiar figure to student and doctor alike.

As I look back, the matter for amazement is not that the drugs and medicines industry as represented by the Association of the British Pharmaceutical Industry (ABPI) was up in arms about the idea of a 'limited list' but that the BMA and the Royal College of General Practitioners decided to support it. They decided to make a stand on their interpretation of a lofty Hippocratic principle – the inalienable duty of doctors at all times to offer what they regarded as the best possible treatment to their patients – in this case presumably regardless of cost to the public purse or of the effectiveness of the remedy.

This in the context of the range of useless preparations currently being paid for from public funds was ludicrous. But it also was a tactic which carried with it the certainty that should ABPI and the BMA lose the argument, they would suffer a painful and very public fall. In due course, that was exactly what happened.

As far as I was concerned, the following weeks were extremely fraught. The dispute between myself and the BMA became public and my first attempt to produce a list of medicines set out under 'generic' not 'trade' names without help from outside the DHSS failed miserably. Meanwhile the ABPI invested in a tendentious national advertising campaign which claimed that the system as it existed was in the best interests of everyone.

But if I had lost a battle, my opponents had certainly not won the war. I decided to go over the heads of the BMA's negotiators and to write to each of the 81,000 doctors in the country explaining what I was trying to achieve. When it became clear that there was by no means unanimous support from the profession for the BMA line, and a powerful leader in "The Times" entitled "Prescribing Propaganda" appeared which backed my plan, the tide turned.

After this, things began to go smoothly and we made swift progress. I had no difficulty in finding experts in the various aspects of therapeutics who were delighted to help prepare what finally came to be called the 'selected' rather than the 'limited' list. Having held our first meeting on 13 January 1985 and sitting almost daily, we had finished the work on 6th February, three weeks later. After a debate in the House of Commons on 18th March, the definitive list of generic medicines which may be prescribed within the National Health Service and paid for from public funds received official blessing. And so with regular amendments to bring it up to date, it remains to the present day.

But that was not quite the end of the story. Some days later when I spoke on a different topic at the Royal Society of Medicine I met a hostile reception from a minority of the audience. The final round of the battle was fired on 17th April at the next meeting of the Standing Medical Advisory Committee - one of the more portentous of the groups which gives counsel to the CMO. A minute on the "limited list" was challenged and I as Chairman was invited to resign. My heart need not have missed a beat! – for this proposal received not a shred of support from anyone.

From the outcome of what must now seem a silly controversy Ministers learned two lessons about the new CMO: he was not in the lap of the British Medical Association and, when the need arose, he was prepared to stand up to unpleasant public controversy.

The Rebirth of Public Health

During my period as CMO, two major initiatives in the development of health policy took place which as I write almost twenty years later can be seen to have put 'public health'[19] back fairly and squarely on the map of human affairs in Britain and the English speaking world abroad.

These were the 'Inquiry into the Future Development of the Public Health Function – Public Health in England' which I chaired and which reported in January 1988, and the national health strategy 'The Health of the Nation' announced in Parliament by John Major as a Green Paper shortly before I stepped down in 1991. While historians may correctly point out that both of these initiatives owed a debt to such archetypal figures as John Simon and David Lloyd George, by the time I arrived in Whitehall in 1983, current events were pointing to an urgent need for a reconsideration and further development in this field.

In the early 1980's the requirement for a review of public health arose for several different reasons. The first was, that a response was needed to criticisms following Public Inquiries into two serious outbreaks of communicable disease in hospitals run by the government – the massive epidemic of salmonella food poisoning at the Stanley Royal mental hospital in Wakefield in 1984 (approximately 400 cases with 20 deaths) and the smaller but just as lethal outbreak of legionellosis a year later due to contaminated spray inhaled by patients and their relatives from a tank on the roof of the new District General Hospital at Stafford (101 cases with 20 deaths).

Both public enquiries pointed to 'a decline in available medical expertise in environmental health and the control of communicable

---

[19] Defined as 'the science and art of preventing disease, prolonging life, and promoting health through organised efforts of society'. See 'Public Health in England'. London. HMSO 1988. Chair. Sir Donald Acheson.

disease'. In the 1980s an even greater concern was the occurrence of a steadily increasing number of cases of AIDS. The containment of this previously unknown and universally fatal infection due to a retrovirus transmitted by sexual intercourse and by blood and blood products, would require innovative policies and a strong public health sector.

But there were also administrative reasons for change which arose from an unfortunate omission from Sir Roy Griffiths "Inquiry into the Management of the NHS", his recommendations having particular force as he had been appointed personally by the Prime Minister, Sir John Major to improve the efficiency of the National Health Service. [20]

In creating a management model for the NHS, Sir Roy Griffiths solution was to transfer in principle, the system which he had found to work so well in his capacity as Chief Executive of Sainsbury's national chain of supermarkets. He proposed, rightly to my mind, to replace the rather flaccid existing NHS system of 'consensus management' in the various Health Authorities[1] by a more decisive arrangement where in each Authority one person, the general manager, clearly vested as such, would be responsible for taking action. These managers would be supported in their 'general management function' by experts in the 'finance', 'personnel', and 'estates' functions as well as by a clinician and a nurse.[21]

---

[20] EDA was well versed in the vagaries of administration within the NHS. Prior to being appointed as CMO he had chaired the Southampton and South West Hampshire Health Authority where he had experienced 'consensus management'. He was also a member of the Wessex Regional Health Authority, and had been a member of the Hampshire Health Authority.

[21] Ibid.

At first, for a period which extended over some difficult months, the Griffiths Report created a situation from which there appeared to be nowhere for doctors with skills in public health to go.[22] But when with the enthusiastic support of the Secretary of State, Norman Fowler, the Inquiry into the Future Development of the Public Health Function was set up and subsequently implemented in 1998, this omission was rectified. The Report required amongst other recommendations that every District and Region should appoint a named leader of what had now become, to match Sir Roy's other managerial tasks, known as the 'public health function' who should be known as the Director of Public Health. And so it remains today.

The epidemic of HIV/Aids, BSE and other infectious diseases which led to a new emphasis on the speciality of Public Health had even wider consequences. They brought about a reappraisal of the relationship to health of health services. Under the leadership of the newly elected Prime Minister, Sir John Major, this led to the creation of a National Health Strategy entitled The Health of the Nation which covered not only behavioural factors such as smoking and alcohol but poverty, poor housing and atmospheric pollution.

---

[22] The post of Medical Officer of Health in the Local Authorities had been abolished in 1974 following a reorganisation of health services.

CHAPTER 10
The Seven Plagues of Egypt

When on my first day in the office Henry Yellowlees had briefed me about the CMO job, he told me that most of my time was likely to be taken up dealing with two subjects: the never ending problems of the NHS, and acting as 'go-between' for Ministers in their various negotiations with the BMA. The 'wider health' including smoking, alcohol abuse, cancer screening and immunisation could probably be dealt with on a one-day a week basis. As for the various infections – influenza, measles, tubercolosis and the like – these in his time had rarely caused problems requiring his personal attention. In the autumn of 1983, when this conversation took place, neither of us could have guessed that events shortly to befall would shatter this perspective for the foreseeable future.

On my arrival in Whitehall, a handful of cases of a mysterious new disease soon to be labelled with the acronym 'AIDs'[23] had already occurred in Amsterdam and San Francisco among gay men. But these had not yet been shown to be due to an infection and their significance was uncertain. Soon two developments were to occur which changed that forever. The first, in 1984, was the discovery that AIDs was in fact due to a retrovirus – HIV – and likely to prove incurable. The second, an even greater bombshell, erupted the following year. I heard from Robert Redford, a colleague in Washington at the Walter Reed Military Institute, that in American soldiers a few of the early cases had been due to infection during <u>vaginal</u> not <u>anal</u> intercourse with an HIV positive person.

---

[23] 'AIDs' is the acronym for the Auto Immune Deficiency Syndrome due to the Human Immunodeficiency Virus (HIV) which destroys the body's defences against infection.

Perhaps due to wishful thinking I did not at first grasp the full implications of this. But the defining moment was not long delayed. It occurred early in the following year and came from a different continent. A package marked 'Urgent, for CMO's personal attention' arrived by messenger from the Foreign and Commonwealth Office across the road. This confirmed as correct, rumours which were circulating of a disaster engulfing parts of Africa. In Zambia, and as I heard later, also in Uganda, HIV was spreading like wildfire in the general population. In some places few adults other than the elderly survived and it was proving difficult to find people to bury the dead. A generation of orphaned children was beginning to appear.

I was horrified. If this could happen in Africa what would an apparently identical virus do in Britain? Having decided that it would be folly to assume that in the UK HIV/AIDs would continue to be confined almost exclusively to gay men, I sought an urgent appointment with my political boss Norman Fowler, the Secretary of State for Health. Norman's reaction was one of deep concern and for the rest of my time in Whitehall, with his unfailing encouragement and support, I was able to give the AIDs epidemic a place close to the top of my priorities.

Almost twenty years later as I write these words, although Britain has so far suffered less from HIV/AIDs than any other European country with colonial links to Africa, there are no grounds for complacency. Globally the epidemic continues to evolve and has by no means reached its peak. No preventative vaccine is yet in sight, and although drugs now available can control symptoms for many years, they remain beyond the pocket of all but the wealthy and insured and involve a complicated regime. In the meantime, in Britain, in recent years an ominous upward trend in the numbers of HIV infections due to vaginal intercourse has once again become apparent particularly in London as people have forgotten the warnings.

As if HIV/AIDs was not enough, in my term of office, Britain was struck by another previously unknown but completely different fatal disease – BSE (bovine spongiform encephalomyelitis) which is caused by eating food contaminated with offal from infected cattle. In addition, quite apart from salmonellosis, two other seemingly obscure infections – legionellosis (Legionnaire's Disease) and listeriosis were responsible for outbreaks of illness sufficient to cause public alarm and to reach the ears of Parliament.

But at a safe distance and in retrospect even plague and pestilence can have a lighter side! Two such occasions were when I received an envelope marked, as if in a James Bond movie, 'Immediate, for CMO's Eyes Only' led initially to action just short of pandemonium – but fortunately were both resolved with a happy outcome. The first related to the discovery of a perfectly preserved corpse in the vault of an ancient London church which had been exposed accidentally by students researching the art of 18th century silver coffin lids. To the horror of all concerned, the body in question displayed the unmistakable marks of the rash of smallpox. The other event, scarcely less alarming was the finding of two phials, one marked Pasteurella Pestis – the microbe of bubonic plague and the other Variola, 1952 (the date of the last outbreak of smallpox in England) in the refrigerators in the laboratory of a London Teaching Hospital. Both of these specimens were found standing immediately adjacent to the technicians' milk and sandwiches!

The phials having been flown urgently under escort to the U.S. National Institute of Health in Atlanta, Georgia, in those days, the only laboratory in the Western world equipped to deal with smallpox, we awaited the outcome with bated breath. Although in both specimens electron microscopy confirmed the presence of the characteristic brick shaped particles of the smallpox virus, these fortunately proved to be inactive. This came as a relief, as the students in the meantime had dispersed on holiday to various unknown destinations on the Mediterranean coast.

'Don't Die of Ignorance': the Government's Response to HIV/AIDs

As has often been the case over the centuries in other epidemics, the discovery that the mysterious condition "AIDs" was in fact due to an infection, led at first to alarm amounting almost to panic. In this case it was not the Jews who in times gone by had so often been the target for irrational attacks who were blamed, but the gay community which became the focus for a punitive response. One extreme proposal in the early days came from an MP who should have known better. His view was that AIDs sufferers should be quarantined permanently in a guarded enclosure on the Isle of Wight. More worrying to us in DHSS, were stories about public discrimination against gay men who had been evicted from their lodgings or refused entry to restaurants.

As far as HIV/Aids was concerned, a few cases of what was already seen as a fatal virus infection associated with infected blood and sexual intercourse had already occurred prior to my appointment. I decided that the implications of the infection was so serious and our knowledge so limited that I should seek expert advice as soon as possible. The expert advisory group on Aids (EAGA) was set up and having met seven times in 1985 and regularly thereafter, it made a series of recommendations which led to more effective control of HIV/Aids within the UK, than in any other country that had links with the African continent.

The authoritative advice of EAGA led to a secure understanding of how the retrovirus was and was not spread which stemmed the risk of mass hysteria. In DHSS, we found ourselves dealing with a seemingly endless series of questions not only on these points but on worries about possible cross infection from butchers, bakers, waiters and even ticket collectors.

In 1985, it became clear that our current approach in the Department to deal with each of these crises as they arose, was no longer tenable. Instead what was needed was to take the bull by the horns and with the help of expert advice[24] make available to everyone in the country a frank and full explanation of the facts – how HIV is and is not spread. I was able to advise the public that HIV does not pass from a close contact as occurs in the tube in rush hour or in the cinema nor in food or water but that it did spread or could spread during sexual intercourse with an infected person without a condom or by infected blood during a transfusion. Although this would inevitably involve distributing explicit information about sex which some people might find offensive, that could not be helped. When I put this proposal to Norman Fowler, whatever concerns he may have had privately about the effect approving such a campaign might have on his future political career, he set these aside and subject to one condition gave the 'Don't Die of Ignorance' Campaign his enthusiastic support.

---

[24] The Expert Advisory Group on Aids provided the scientific advice on which the UK's policies were based.

The stipulation on which Norman Fowler's consent to the '<u>Don't Die of Ignorance</u>' Campaign depended, was to lead me down a path which I suspect no CMO has trodden before or since. It also occasioned one of the most memorable experiences of my career. I was to consult and try to gain, at least the acquiescence, if not the approval of four key national figures: none other than the Archbishop of Canterbury, the Cardinal of Westminster, the Moderator of the Free Churches and the Chief Rabbi. Having first searched unavailingly for a twinkle in Norman Fowler's eye, I began to realise this was not a joke but a serious proposition. Some hope, I thought to myself! Nor were my spirits restored by the mirthful expressions on the faces of my office staff when I asked them to make the necessary appointments. Even though almost twelve years have elapsed, as the meetings were in strict confidence it would be wrong to go into detail about who said what. But there can be no harm in writing about the substance.

The memory I have is not, as I had feared, of a series of tirades on sin, repentance and judgement. Far from that, the four religious leaders' concerns related exclusively to the unfolding tragedy of the epidemic and its increasing toll of untimely deaths among young people and children. As for my own rôle, which included giving explicit advice about risk reduction on TV and radio, they had nothing but support and encouragement. I had feared that in particular my promotion of the use of condoms as a prophylactic against the spread of infection would prove controversial. In the event, neither on that occasion or later did I receive any criticism from anyone including the Cardinal about my promotion of condoms. Although all of them taught that sexual fidelity within marriage was the golden rule and some held that homosexual intercourse was an abomination, it turned out that they were united in respecting the intentions of the Government's campaign to protect health and united in admiration for my energetic persistence.

The "bottom line" was that, whatever reservations they might have about the details, none of the four religious leaders would preach against the 'Don't Die of Ignorance' campaign, nor any part of it – nor if they could help it, would their clergy. From that day to this, all of them and their successors have been as good as their word.

Fortunately for the United Kingdom, Norman Fowler's contribution to the control of HIV, led to two sets of policies which had a major impact. The first was the campaign using radio, television and the press to give explicit information about the means of transmission of the virus which led to the advice "if you don't stick to one partner, use a condom." Secondly, to inform the public that the infection was not limited to homosexual men. In the process of making this point it was necessary to explain to the public the distinction between vaginal and anal intercourse. Although this temporarily was too much for the Prime Minister, Margaret Thatcher to contemplate, with the support of Lord Whitelaw, the Deputy Prime Minister, she was prepared to adopt an accurately phrased account which was duly used in the national public education campaign 'Don't Die of Ignorance'.

As far as Norman Fowler was concerned, that was by no means the end of the story. It was he, who shortly afterwards had the courage to introduce another policy which although controversial at the time as aiding and abetting an illegal practice, has I believe, also been a significant factor in containing the epidemic in Britain. This was to authorise the creation of a chain of distribution points throughout the National Health Service where at public expense, intravenous (I.V.)

drug abusers could and still can, obtain clean work's (clean work's – is the slang word used for equipment including needles and syringes used by people who inject themselves with heroin etc) in exchange for their old needles and condoms and advice on safe sex to this day. Nearly twenty years later IVDA's contribute a minute part of the British epidemic.

But the implications of the 'Don't Die of Ignorance' Campaign, which I hoped would include a leaflet drop to every household in the land, were such that they would require the consent of the Government as a whole. That this, in the event, did not prove insurmountable was due not only to Norman Fowler's support but to the efforts of two other outstanding public servants, Sir Robert Armstrong and Lord Whitelaw. As Secretary to the Cabinet, Sir Robert was the most senior civil servant in the land and was also the person to whom I, as CMO was accountable. Lord Whitelaw's support as Deputy Prime Minister would also be essential if our campaign was to obtain, as it must sooner or later, the approval of the Prime Minister. Thanks to their efforts and advice Margaret Thatcher agreed, Lord Whitelaw's help having been - contrary to what might have been expected from an elderly Tory grandee – decisive.

"Pep it up, and don't beat about the bush", I remember him saying, *"You won't shock me! I'm an old soldier and know all about this sort of thing."*

And so with the help of a detailed survey of the sexual habits of the British people conducted on behalf of the Government by the Wellcome Institute to help us predict future trends, we did!

At the first meeting of the Whitelaw Committee in November 1985, I witnessed the most effective piece of Chairmanship of my life whether in Whitehall or elsewhere. Driving the other members – almost exclusively of Cabinet rank – like a flock of chickens, within the space of and hour and a half, William Whitelaw had got agreement for:

- a universal leaflet drop to every household explaining how HIV spread,
- free time on TV and radio for health messages,

and

- a new set of newspaper and poster advertisements.

At the same time he stamped firmly on the idea of an 'AIDs public education council', which he declared would simply cause delay in actions we all agreed were urgently necessary, and also upon the notion that immigrants should be screened for HIV at the ports.

The first of the Whitelaw recommendations was in my view the most sensitive. After all a person who was shocked by a radio or television message could turn it off and even a full-page advertisement in a newspaper could be ignored. But a leaflet in an envelope marked "Important Information for Your Health" dropped through every letterbox in the land, be the occupant priest, parent or prostitute, was another matter. In fact, from more than twenty million leaflets delivered there emerged only one complaint – from a Member of Parliament who returned his leaflet unopened with an abusive note addressed personally to me.

The culmination of the 'Don't Die of Ignorance' Campaign was the publication of the explicit full-page advertisements recommended by Whitelaw (including the headline "Stick to one partner; if you can't, use a condom") simultaneously on Sunday in all the national newspapers.

This, some of my friends felt, would prove to be 'a bridge too far' not least because of the wide circulation English newspapers have outside the U.K., for example, in Ireland and on the continent. I remember vividly, the moment early that Sunday morning when the telephone woke me up. This must be the first of an avalanche of complaints about the disgusting advertisements desecrating the Sabbath day, I thought. In fact to my relief it was simply a neighbour saying the paperboy had delivered two papers, ours as well as his, to him. He thought the advertisement was good stuff, 'if a bit racy', as did his mother aged 81.

As it turned out, there were no complaints about those advertisements on that day or subsequently.

There were however one or two hiccoughs along the way. The first was when the British Medical Association with the best intentions announced that people who had had more than one sex partner in the past two years should not donate blood. This advice was withdrawn just in time to prevent the collapse of the transfusion system for want of donors. The second was when the names of two doctors with HIV were leaked to the News of the World. I sought an injunction from the High Court to protect them. The judge accepted my advice but the News of the World responded by publishing a scurrilous article about me in their newspaper in 1987.

But that was by no means the end of the matter which rumbled on for several weeks with widespread further press coverage. On the one hand statements were made that doctors particularly surgeons had the right to know if their patients were HIV positive, and on the other hand proposals emerged from elevated circles of Government, that doctors should be subjected to regular compulsory screening. Finally, a strict new set of rules from the GMC to guide members of the medical profession, settled the matter once and for all, and I, marvellous to relate, was congratulated for getting the GMC 'to crack the whip at last' and issue such a firm statement.

Princess Diana

Perhaps overshadowed by her tragic later life, Diana's rôle during the early years of the HIV/AIDs epidemic seems to have been forgotten. Yet the simple, direct and let it be said, fearless example of this largely untutored young woman, by allowing herself to be photographed embracing people of all ages infected by HIV – babies, children and adults – probably had more influence in dispelling irrational fears and bringing HIV/AIDs in from the cold than all the Government's leaflets and advertisements put together.

Neither was Diana's work on AIDs the 'flash in the pan' that might have been expected if she had simply been seeking publicity. It was substantial over several years. I was fortunate to meet her on a number of occasions, for example, when she opened the new HIV/AIDs ward at the Middlesex Hospital in April 1985 and five and a half years later when I was present at the opening of 'Positively Women's[25] new HQ in Islington. I know also that in the intervening years she was a regular visitor – often late at night to avoid the Press – at the Mildmay Hospital in Hackney and at the 'London Lighthouse'.

Here is an excerpt from my diary about Diana:

3rd Dec 1990

My day started with a visit to Positively Women's new HQ in Islington. Princess Diana 'opened' it though without speech or plaque. This beautiful and dignified young woman simply by being

---

[25] A charitable organisation for HIV Positive women.

there and talking quietly in turn to each of the women transformed the occasion. Sheila G. thin but very cheerful made a marvellous speech in her strong Glasgow accent without notes. Her baby, now two years old, turns out <u>not</u> to have been infected during pregnancy and is HIV negative. I also met two smiling Ugandan women and a sad looking ex-Edinburgh drug abuser. The place was full of nice people and we were met at the door by a young man with a pink Mohican coxcomb. Incongruously, the house itself is part of a listed 18th century terrace with a magnificently carved oak fireplace.

AIDs in the 'New World'

During 1987 I visited the United States about AIDs twice. In the first, in January, I accompanied Norman Fowler and we visited New York, San Francisco and Washington. In the second, in October, his successor John Moore and I revisited New York, and had the opportunity to look at the situation there in greater depth.

What we were to find on these visits was not one catastrophe but two. First, tens possibly hundreds of thousands of infected people in New York, San Francisco and other parts of the USA, mostly under 40 years old and all of whom would die within the next few years. Norman and I were deeply moved, indeed harrowed by what we saw. And second, at the Federal level from Ronald Reagan down, a state of complete psychological denial even seemingly to the very existence of the HIV/AIDs epidemic. Hand-in-hand with this attitude which a charitable view might hold stemmed from the Puritanism of the Pilgrim Fathers, went blindness to the need of any public explanation of the illness or of how to protect oneself against it. However, at a local level, as we were to find in San Francisco and in New York, good work was being done.

The occasion of the second visit to New York after an interval of nine months gave me the opportunity to review the creeping AIDs disaster in that city.

> *The position in New York City has progressed inexorably since January – now 320 cases appearing a month with 60% of the Bellevue Hospital's beds occupied by AIDs and perhaps 500,000 people infected. We visited the Haarlem Hospital at 135th Street. A ward full of AIDs-stricken children, some abandoned and with nowhere to go… Few are expected to reach puberty. To say that the self-chosen devotion of those looking after these doomed children was edifying is an understatement.*

Everywhere, the fact that on two occasions Conservative Cabinet Ministers from Britain had been sufficiently interested in HIV/AIDs to cross the Atlantic was a matter for wonderment. And everywhere, we were accompanied by a vast retinue of the Press. At the personal level both Norman Fowler and John Moore, as I was myself, were harrowed and distressed by the wards filled with young men and children sick and dying of a fatal disease.

But as Norman Fowler and I stepped wearily down from the plane at Heathrow on our return from Washington, we found that while we were away a storm had been gathering. The Prime Minister, Mrs Thatcher, had apparently associated herself publicly with an almost crazy moralistic speech by Anderton, the Head Constable of Manchester. In this speech, he had claimed divine inspiration for referring to gay men and I.V. drug abusers as a '*scum floating on a sea of corruption*'. Norman Fowler's reaction was robust and a great credit to him. He said, that even if some other members of the Cabinet might share this view he was convinced his approach was right. He did not really care what others thought and would continue on his course regardless. And so he did. Meanwhile the storm quickly blew itself out and may have been due to a misunderstanding.

We then went to Belgium where the epidemic in heterosexuals affected both sexes equally. Was this due to a different strain of virus in the Belgian Congo?

28th February 1987

Aids continues to dominate everything. Last night there was a TV programme in which Norman and I both appeared. A proposal from one member of the panel that there should be universal testing and quarantine got little support.

30th May 1987

Yesterday news came from our Washington Embassy that President Reagan is to make a statement tomorrow in which he will express the hope that in future people will agree to be tested for HIV on admission to hospital, before marriage, on attending sexually transmitted disease clinics or pregnancy. Or on being sent to prison . In my view there is a substantial downside to these suggestions - unless confidentiality is strictly adhered to. This was not mentioned.

October 1987

Debate on HIV/Aids in New York and later in Paris. Speeches at both are made by John Moore who had at that time replaced Norman Fowler as Health & Social Services Secretary.

The first World Summit on HIV/Aids was held in London in 1988, jointly sponsored by WHO and the UK government. 120 ministers were present including a representative of the Holy See who could not accept the value of condoms. Later, I held a meeting with Prudential Insurance Company on HIV/Aids. Instead of trying to identify high risk groups and load their premiums they have decided that everyone who wants to take out a policy for more than £100,000,00 should be required to take a HIV test and they would not ask any questions regarding sexual orientation.

Twenty years later after the early cases of HIV in the UK, the measures taken to try to reduce the spread of HIV have stood the country in good stead. In 2004 the number of cases while not as low as occurs in the Scandinavian countries, is lower than any other country with a colonial history in Africa and the epidemic due to intravenous drug abuse has been avoided.

The World Summit on AIDs in London, January 1988

In many ways the culmination of my work on AIDs was the 'World Summit' which took place in London in January 1988 and was organised jointly with the World Health Organisation (WHO) and hosted by the United Kingdom Government. It was a resounding success with an unparalleled attendance of more than 120 Ministers and 149 delegates – including one from the Holy See – from all corners of the globe.

Unlike most international conferences, the audience's attention was riveted throughout. There were two striking aspects in addition to first class presentations and organisation. The first, was the standard of the contributions of Ministers from the various countries – none of whom made political points but updated their country's epidemiological position and gave frank accounts of the specific cultural problems. I remember in particular Sierra Leone – the Minister fearful of the arrival of the virus because of the tradition of many sexual partners – 'an area between marriage and prostitution' which he explained accounted for a substantial part of the distribution of the wealth of the country; and Lesotho where the mineworkers away from their families not only made use of prostitutes but of homosexual relationships.

But the choice of the contributors of scientific papers was one of the best features. A Kenyan lady in full African dress, spoke in perfect English about the details of her health education campaign among Nairobi prostitutes – the majority of whom were already HIV positive; and an Australian Aborigine health visitor described the acceptance and commitment she had obtained from her own people – by using a colour scheme on her posters which they could identify with.

These contributions must have had an impact on strengthening the resolve of other Ministers to deal likewise with the risks of disadvantaged and alienated people whether among the Greenland Eskimos or the South American shanty dwellers. My own contribution which focussed on the unpleasant details of risky behaviours associated with transmission of the virus was received not in disgust but with enthusiasm.

The conference ended with the 'London Declaration' which went much further than the platitudes which often conclude international conferences, and, although the USSR and China abstained, otherwise I received almost universal commitment. The Declaration is based on the following principles: the containment and reduction of the spread of HIV should be based on accurate and freely exchanged scientific information; the protection of human rights and dignity; and by education, persuasion and support rather than condemnation and punishment.[26]

Aids Ethics at the Elysēe Palace and at WHO

In May 1989, when I arrived in Paris from Geneva for the first meeting of the French Committee on 'The Ethical Aspects of Aids/HIV' I was both tired and jaded. Not only had I been away from my London office for ten days attending the World Health Assembly, but the only English newspaper available in the plane – the 'Independent' – featured a story about an unfortunate rift between my boss Kenneth Clarke and myself before I left. It alleged that following a threat of resignation on my part, Kenneth had had to think again about the membership of the newly created National Health Service Policy Board and include me as ex officio as CMO on it as a member.

At the World Health Assembly, the massive problems of global ill health had put this petty backstairs gossip in its proper perspective. Since my first attendance there in 1984, as UK Head of Delegation perhaps the most important achievement of WHO, had been to develop the radical idea of 'primary health care,' and get it accepted by many of the poorest countries. This proposes that top priority should be given - not as had previously been the case, to the construction, at great expense of European style hospitals, only of use to the minority within walking distance, but the provision for everyone of basic essentials such as clean water, shelter and immunisation. With this should go hand, in hand the empowerment of women as the key agents to promote personal hygiene, contraception and nutrition within the family.

---

[26] A major factor in the triumph of the so-called 'liberal consensus' rather than a punitive approach was due to the work at WHO of the late Dr Jonathan Mann at WHO. Dr Mann died tragically in an aircraft accident in 1990.

Although at the Assembly, as CMO I was formally Head of the UK Delegation, I would have achieved nothing without the help of John Sankey, the British Ambassador in Geneva, and his staff of professional diplomats.

In view of the ongoing crisis in the Middle East, it is worth recounting that almost twenty five years ago in 1989, the issue which split the World Health Assembly and led to seemingly endless debate stemmed from the same roots. It was the question of the admission of the 'State of Palestine' to full membership. These discussions took place in the presence of a familiar figure – Yassar Arafat – looking ageless – and wearing his characteristic headdress.   As the delegations were seated alphabetically, the UK, together with the USA, and the USSR, were close to the back of the hall next to the area for official visitors. These included on this occasion, Mr Arafat, with whom, as he spoke English, I used to exchange greetings and pleasantries.   But on the substantive issue of Palestine's Membership of the Assembly, it was John Sankey, the professional diplomat, not I, who found the magic formula on which all could agree – the deferment of the decision until next year!

Guest of Honour at the Elysée

The meeting on the first morning of France's 'Aids and Ethics' conference proved to be tiresome. I found myself co-opted as 'rapporteur' of a group dealing with the social, economic and legal problems of HIV, which meant I had the task of submitting a summary paper later in the day. At first I thought I would have to give up and say I simply could not manage it – the issues were complex; my notes copious; my brain did not seem to be working properly and attendants kept interrupting me to clear away coffee cups, glasses etc. But in the end it all came together in the form of a heavily amended script for delivery in the afternoon session under the chairmanship of none other than President Mitterand himself.

In the event, partly because Mitterand was half an hour late, the tension continued to build and became almost unbearable. My talk turned out not to be a flop but was a success, and I found my English being complimented both for clarity of language and content. My reward was to be invited to join François Mitterand and to sit at his right hand for the remainder of the day – a man who although of diminutive stature dominated proceedings and came away with all the laurels.

Although his approach was friendly and informal, François Mitterand's deep concern about the tragedy of the HIV/Aids epidemic was obvious from the outset.

"One episode of sexual intercourse, one swap of a syringe and needle are" - as he put it – *"terrifyingly sufficient to transmit Aids. We must all think of our responsibilities"*.

It was his use of the word 'we' which was so riveting. His message was that HIV/Aids is a problem for everyone whatever their station in life, President or commoner, in France or beyond.

Reflecting on the speech afterwards, I hoped that the personal concern of France's Head of State expressed in such intimate terms and addressed as it seemed to each one of us would strengthen resolve for HIV/Aids to be taken seriously everywhere.

The HIV/AIDs epidemic in Britain Today

That tragically was not the end of the story. It is proving to have been only the beginning. During the last five years the increase in the number of cases of HIV infection has been steeper than at any time since statistics became available in 1985. By the end of 2002 there were approximately 50,000 people in the UK living with HIV. Admittedly, treatment now available has extended the lives of infected people but there is another side to that coin which is worrying. Drugs currently available do not cure the infection by the retrovirus but only suppress it. What is more the treatment is complex, it has to be continued indefinitely and unless taken meticulously does not guarantee that the patient is at all times non infectious to others.

Alongside the year on year increase in the reports of HIV which in 2002 reached 4750 there are similar increases in new infections with gonorrhea. Taken together, these ominous portents suggest that young people have forgotten the lessons of the 1980s and have recently become more inclined to risk unprotected sex.

The geography of HIV within the UK is remarkable. Although no area has escaped completely, more than half of the 50,000 people known to be infected live in London. Particularly perplexing is the recent sharp rise in the number of HIV cases where infection has been in the continent of Africa. Whatever the political implications of that fact eventually turn out to be, London residents urgently need to have the central message of the previous Aids campaign put before them again. On TV, Radio and in public advertisements the warning should go out: 'Stick to one partner, if you don't, use a condom!'

Most people's concept of the meaning of the word 'epidemic' is based on illness like influenza or food poisoning where the outbreak begins or ends within a few weeks. Where people unknowingly carry the HIV/Aids retrovirus for years, the word has totally different implications. In Britain, we should be thinking in terms of an epidemic with a perspective not of years but of decades where if the infection is not to become endemic – a semi permanent feature of our society as did syphilis and tuberculosis – we need a longer term strategy than is apparent today. In 1986, the issue of testing for HIV at the ports was considered and turned down as much on the basis of practicability as on any other grounds. It seems increasingly unlikely that HIV within the UK will reach levels experienced in Africa, Brazil, India and Thailand.

Edwina

Edwina Currie's career in Whitehall rather like a visitation of Halley's Comet, was brief but spectacular. Although her appointment was as a junior minister, in this case it came straight from 10 Downing Street when Mrs Thatcher had discovered that with one other exception she, as Prime Minister was the only woman in government. In the DHSS we looked forward to her arrival as likely to enliven our routine. This it certainly did.

I have a clear recollection of my first meeting with Edwina. As was customary with a new Minister I made an appointment to go down to her office to meet her. The young attractive brunette behind the desk stood up with a bright smile, walked to the table in the middle of the room, hitched her skirt above her knees, crossed her legs and offered me a place beside her at the table.

"You will have already noted CMO that I have two nice legs", she said, *"you should also know that I have two excellent university degrees!"*

Edwina's difficulty was that, in spite of all these helpful attributes she was at times wayward about accepting advice. During the salmonella – egg crisis she made the mistake of giving an interview to a journalist from her home at the weekend without proper briefing. The impression she gave, that the majority of eggs might be infected, when the truth was closer to 1 in a 1000, knocked the bottom out of the market. For a time, while hens continued to lay and eggs could not be sold, stocks piled up and had to be tipped down mine shafts or otherwise destroyed. Tearful deputations of farmers arrived in the Department. Bankruptcies may have ensued.

A second occasion when Edwina had misunderstood her brief and made a broadcast was perhaps even more unfortunate. She allowed herself to say, that cervical cancer was due to 'women sleeping around'. The truth is, that while one factor in the causation of cervical cancer is a virus spread by sexual intercourse, it may sometimes originate from the male partner who has been 'sleeping around' and be passed to a female who has not. Subsequently, I tried to correct the misunderstanding myself in a further broadcast.

Mad Cow Disease

Bovine Spongiform Encephalomyelitis, or BSE as everyone now calls it, is a fatal disease of cattle due to what is rather pompously known as an 'unconventional transmissible agent' or 'prion'. The epidemic in the 1980's was caused by the introduction of 'meat and bone meal' in cattle food or 'MBM', a product made by the cannibalistic practice of supplementing cattle food by grinding up the carcases of cows. This unpleasant idea came into vogue because animals fed in this way fattened more quickly, than those fed exclusively on grass and hay, their natural foods. Tragically, the prion in MBM, in addition to infecting cattle was subsequently to cross the species barrier and spread to humans who had eaten infected products. At the time of writing, approximately 200 people within the UK, mostly in the prime of life have died of the related disease 'new variant Creutzfeld Jakob Disease' or 'nv CJD' – as it is commonly called. The fact that the epidemic nv CJD now seems to be in decline is the first gleam of hope in an otherwise appalling scene.

As I was Chief Medical Officer when BSE was identified in March 1988, I was involved in the public health response to it until my retirement from that role in 1991. Subsequently my actions were scrutinised by Lord Phillips in his Public Inquiry into the epidemic published in 2000. While I received some praise, I was also criticised in a way which in my view seems to rely heavily on hindsight.

The first news I had of the BSE epidemic in cattle came simultaneously from two sources on 3rd March 1988. A note from Derek Andrews, the Permanent Secretary of the Ministry of Agriculture, Food and Fisheries (MAFF) described the epidemic which had started in 1986 in general terms and asked for advice. The second from the doctor who was my liaison officer with MAFF was a good deal more informative. This brought the news that Andrews' admirable plan to control the epidemic by making the disease notifiable so that the affected cattle could be destroyed had already been turned down by the Treasury. This was because of the costs of compensation to farmers that such a policy would create.

A brilliant research study at the National Agricultural Institute at Weybridge had already pinpointed the cause of the disease. BSE was due to the recent introduction of a novel way of speeding up the fattening of cattle for market. Unfortunately this involved the cannibalistic feeding of rations enriched with 'meat and bone meal' (MBM) derived from the carcasses of their own species and other livestock.

A quote from my personal diary at that time reads:

11ᵗʰ March 1988

We have another plague in Egypt. A year or so ago it became clear that a new spongiform encephalophathy has appeared particularly in dairy herds... A brilliant epidemiological study suggests it is due to the use of tallow derived from brain fat in animal feed... The 'virus' is probably already in the food chain. If we are dealing with the scrapie agent in sheep there is no evidence that this has infected man by the oral route for at least 100 years. But at present one does not know enough to write off any risk of eating ox brain less than adequately cooked. I am calling an urgent meeting next week.

My judgement was and still remains that it would have been quite wrong for me to rush in to a public warning without first taking urgent expert advice. The epidemic was at that time exclusively in cattle and the precedent of scrapie in sheep suggested the agent might be harmless to humans. Since public health warnings may affect the behaviour of millions of people they must be based on unequivocal expert scientific advice and sound reasoning.

That my instinct had been correct was borne out when even the group of veterinarians and other experts I had summoned urgently to advise me two weeks later themselves found the issues too difficult to resolve at a single meeting – not least because an early attempt at DNA sequencing of the BSE prions just published in Edinburgh further supported (wrongly as it later turned out) the view that the prion was indeed identical to harmless scrapie. The unprecedented nature of the problem would require the attention of a different group of experts whose experience focussed specifically on animal virology and ecology. The unfortunate price of this was that 'the slaughter and compensation order' had to wait until after the first meeting of the expert committee on 20ᵗʰ June I had urgently set to be chaired by Sir Richard Southwood.

Although the Phillips Inquiry took the view that I personally should have challenged the Treasury's decision to overrule MAFF's recommendation for slaughter three months previously, this seems nonsense as the CMO's role is advisory and includes no executive powers particularly in financial matters. The only possible approach, in theory, would have been for me to seek the help of the Prime Minister, Mrs Thatcher, but in the face of the lack of evidence available at the time such a view puts even the notion of hindsight under strain. In any case, this would probably have been to no avail for even when as described below, Southwood recommended a ban of bovine offal in baby food the Prime Minister was highly sceptical of the need to do this and sent for me for an explanation.

The other criticisms of my response to BSE/CJD crisis can be dealt with quite briefly.

The Phillips Inquiry held, quite rightly in my view, that the Department of Health ought to have undertaken a review of the Southwood Report when it was published in 1989. I agreed with this and had in fact requested such a review. However they chose not to accept my evidence that this had actually been done. My difficulty in convincing the Inquiry, was that the senior official Dr Ed Harris, whose responsibility was to advise me on infectious diseases, and who had undertaken the review, had died and so could not corroborate my evidence. Fortunately Dr Michael Abrams, a close colleague, whose office was adjacent to Dr Harris, has subsequently confirmed that my evidence on this point was correct.

In his report, Sir Richard Southwood did not advise that bovine offal (liver, brain, kidney etc) should be removed from the shops but as a measure of "extreme prudence" that it should be excluded from baby food. He had two reasons for making this exception. First, babies are particularly vulnerable because their immune systems are not fully developed and second, baby food often comprises 100% of their diet. The Phillips Inquiry criticised me for not overruling him, but as he knew far more about this matter than I did, that was not a practical option. In other words, if you get experts to advise and they do a careful job one can't easily overrule them. Ironically, when the Southwood Report was put before the Cabinet, the Prime Minister, herself a mother and a housewife, asked not for a wider ban to be introduced but whether the baby food ban was really necessary and could be set aside. Later, MAFF decided to take the matter into its own hands and implemented a ban on specified beef offal in all food for adults, children and babies alike.

Goodbye to Whitehall

Two important Ministerial changes were to make my final twelve months as CMO the most interesting and productive I experienced as a civil servant. In November 1990, the Thatcher government fell and John Major became Prime Minister, with William Waldegrave as Health Secretary. As my office in Whitehall was directly opposite Downing Street, I had immediate notice of this seismic event. As TV and Radio broadcasts announced the tearful moment, there was a loud cheer from the gathering crowd and a man began to ring a hand bell.

I had got to know John Major well because earlier in his career he had been Minister of Social Security in our own department during the bitter winter of 1986. I was able to show him that due to our shocking national heritage of poorly insulated and unheated housing, the excess mortality in winter in Britain was higher than in the far colder climates of Scandinavia and Central Europe. The winter fuel allowance was the first step in a raft of policies he introduced across Whitehall to deal with this problem and rehabilitate the public housing stock.

John Major's personal background and our easy relations in the department also meant he was open to other ideas. One of these, although radical at the time, was that in spite of its obvious merits, the National Health Service while providing free treatment for a wide range of ailments – be they hernia or haemorrhoids, hypertension or breast cancer – was insufficient on its own to improve the nations health. John abhorred smoking and drinking to excess and was quick to respond to the idea of a national strategy for health, tackling all the main risk factors e.g. diet, housing, transport, smoking and so on.

As Prime Minister, it was John Major who set the seal once and for all on the 'Health of the Nation' strategy by hosting an all day seminar at 'Chequers' his official country residence.

27th April 1991

In the car on the way to Chequers. The leak of the 'Health Strategy' to the press yesterday did not cause much of a negative impact, indeed it turned out to be quite the contrary despite Robin Cook's (at the time 'shadow' Health Secretary) efforts. But the fact that Guy's Hospital is to fire 600 staff to balance their books is causing a major impact which may spoil today's seminar.

Chequer's is a large red-brick house - perhaps 17th century and much extended recently – standing alone in a secluded and sparsely inhabited valley in the Chilterns. It is surprisingly exposed from the road and to my wonderment, such apparently is the strength of England's common law, has a well trodden public foot path across the grounds.

The meeting was in a room with a long table – almost a replica of the cabinet room at No 10 Downing Street. As well as the Prime

Minister and all the Health Ministers, a number of medical and nursing luminaries from the Royal Colleges and the BMA were present. An amusing moment was when Christine Hancock (at that time President of the Royal College of Nursing) found herself explaining how many people who had done badly at school were good at practical (she quickly added) and <u>other</u> tasks – when she remembered the press interest in the PM's extremely meagre O' levels. He roared with laughter and remarked that he was glad she had added 'other'.

In addition to chairing the meeting he acted as host (his wife was not present) and, as ever, his careful courtesy and trouble to talk to everyone and make them feel at home was evident and most impressive.

The seminar was not just constructive but of a very high calibre despite press expectations to the contrary. It not only dealt with the 'Health of the Nation' document including its relationship to WHO's regional strategy for health in Europe but also attempted to predict in general terms how health and healthcare would look in 2000:

- *Aging of the population would continue*
- *The spectrum of disease would remain much the same*
- *Health care workers would remain in short supply and would need to 'retask' at regular intervals*
- *Needs of inner cities should be looked at again*
- *Ethical issues would provide more difficult problems*
- *Genetics would lead to wide insights and new techniques*

At Chequers, there are stained glass windows dedicated to each Prime Minister. From where I was sitting I could see windows to Wilson, Home and Callaghan.

The Health of the Nation 'Roadshow'

A consultative document 'The Health of the Nation' was set before Parliament in June 1991 and for the remainder of the weeks before the summer holidays, William Waldegrave, the new Secretary of State for Health, and I toured the Southern and Western shires with what became know as the 'Roadshow'. In some ways, reminiscent of an Elizabethan 'Progress' we stopped off at various welcoming hospitals in the Southern and Western shires where we did a double act, my part being to explain the facts of health and ill health and his to announce the new portfolio of policies. I remember it as a relaxed occasion in the company of a cultured and highly intelligent country gentleman.

A note of our visit to Bristol tried to put all our recent efforts in perspective:

> *Most of the day spent on the Health Strategy Roadshow's visit to Bristol. It was a success. W.W's speech went well and was also complimented. I put the strategy in the context of the 1871 Public Health Act, the Ministry of Health Act of 1920 and the 1948 Act which set up the NHS. During the discussion someone produced a remarkable supplement of the Times dated 30th September 1937 believe it or not, entitled 'The Health of the Nation'. Chamberlain, who was Prime Minister at the time, was photographed salmon fishing on p2 with a large advertisement by the BMA proposing a 'national general medical service' on p3 which was a step towards the NHS not a wider health strategy.*

In 2004, more than a decade after the publication of the 'Health of the Nation' document by John Major's Conservative Government, the importance of the existence of a national strategy for health has been acknowledged – although without giving credit for its predecessor - by Tony Blair's Labour Administration in 'Saving Lives: our Healthier Nation'. As well as placing more emphasis on socio-economic factors in the genesis of ill health than its predecessor and focussing on the reduction of inequalities as a priority, it identifies four 'killers' for particular attention – cancer; coronary heart disease and stroke; accidents and mental illness and sets targets for each to be met by 2010. Setting aside these differences, the key point which emerges is that an organised effort to sustain and improve health led by government but trying to involve everyone and reaching far beyond the National Health Service seems now to be a permanent feature of the British scene.

For instance, as might be expected if one invites people to do something positive rather than to stop doing something they like it is often more likely to succeed. Thus my suggestion that everyone, and in particular children should eat five portions of fruit or vegetables each day was much more widely accepted than to advise them to stop smoking.

When I was Chief Medical Officer, so much of my energy was used dealing with the crises and events of the day, that it was difficult to imagine that any long term benefits would be achieved. As I look back now, however, some fifteen years later I can see major outcomes which seem likely to be permanent and beneficial. This is the renaissance of public health which has brought with it the ideas that health cannot be achieved by the National Health Service alone but in addition requires a healthy lifestyle, acceptable housing, schools, work places and public transport. Public health as a profession extending beyond medical practitioners is now well established and includes nurses and health visitors and environmental health workers. Directors of public health have now been appointed throughout the country ideally working jointly with the local authorities and the National Health Service. A development which I can take some credit for, is the strengthening of the system of health statistics by the establishment of a central health monitoring unit in Whitehall.

Having retired as CMO on my sixty fifth birthday, I was recalled shortly afterwards by the then Minister of State at the Home Office, Ann Widdecombe to investigate the health of prisoners. As there is already an Inspectorate of Prisons and also a Prison Medical Service this took a good deal of tact. In the process, I visited some 28 prisons all over the country. This is not the occasion where I wish to write a chapter on my prison visits. However, I am happy to put on paper my profound admiration for the work of the custodians often discharging their duties patiently and professionally in the most appalling environment, often in Victorian unmodernised prisons more than a 100 years old.

I wish to make a single point with all the force I can muster. In a system where prisoners may be incarcerated at the opposite end of the country to their homes e.g. a Tyneside man on the Isle of Wight. Public funds should be found to allow the families to visit. Otherwise an additional penalty over and above the sentence of the court without the knowledge of the jury has been exacted. In a sentence of several years, family breakdown due to lack of contact becomes inevitable with all of its implications of further offences. I feel this should be put right as a matter of urgency.

Index

INDEX

INDEX